Mental Health Provider's Guide
to Managed Care

Mental Health Provider's Guide to Managed Care

Industry Insiders Reveal How to Successfully Participate and Profit in Today's System

Leonard Reich

Andrew Kolbasovsky

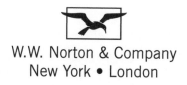

W.W. Norton & Company
New York • London

The content of this book solely reflects the opinions of the authors.

For information about permission to reproduce
selections from this book, write to
Permissions, W. W. Norton & Company, Inc.,
500 Fifth Avenue, New York, NY 10110

Manufacturing by Haddon Craftsmen
Production Manager: Leeann Graham

Library of Congress Cataloging-in-Publication Data

Reich, Leonard Hugh, 1942–
    Mental health provider's guide to managed care / Leonard Reich and
Andrew Kolbasovsky.
        p.   cm.
    "A Norton professional book."
    Includes bibliographical references.
    ISBN 13: 978-0-393-70504-1
    ISBN 10: 0-393-70504-8
    1. Managed mental health care.   2. Psychotherapy-Effect of managed
care on.   I. Kolbasovsky, Andrew.   II. Title.

RC465.6.R45 2007
3 2.2'0425—dc226   2006048265

        ISBN 13: 978-0-393-70504-1
        ISBN 10: 0-393-70504-8

W. W. Norton & Company, Inc., 500 Fifth Avenue, New York, N.Y. 10110
www.wwnorton.com
W. W. Norton & Company Ltd., Castle House, 75/76 Wells St., London W1T 3QT
1 2 3 4 5 6 7 8 9 0

This book is dedicated to my wife, Dr. Tina Reich, for her wisdom and thoughtful professional guidance, and to my four daughters, Briana, Nicole, Rosandra, and Keira, for being such special women.
—Leonard Reich

This book is dedicated to the great joys of my life, my wife, Lia, and my daughters, Juliana and Grace.
—Andrew Kolbasovsky

Contents

Mental Health Provider's Guide to Managed Care

CHAPTER ONE

The Current Environment of Managed Behavioral Health Care

Despite the sometimes negative connotations of working with managed care, the current managed care context offers mental health providers who understand the system wonderful opportunities to develop lasting and financially rewarding practices. Yet, despite this opportunity, many mental health providers have chosen to limit or even eliminate their involvement with managed care, citing reasons such as an insufficient reimbursement rate or an overwhelming amount of required paperwork (Psychotherapy Finances, 2000). While it may be true that the onset of managed care has lowered reimbursement rates for many providers and participation with managed care does involve paperwork, providers who understand how to operate in the managed care environment can greatly increase the number of referrals generated to them while also greatly limiting the amount of time spent on paperwork.

While some providers have preferred to treat only self-paying patients, the reality is that most people in need of mental health services are not able to self-pay for these services and will therefore need to use their insurance coverage. Since most potential patients will need to pay for services through their insurance, the best way for most mental health providers to develop a financially rewarding practice is to develop a relationship with one or more managed care organizations. This book is designed to help you navigate all important facets of working with managed care in order to develop a financially and professionally rewarding relationship. To this end, this book will provide you with practical inside tips on all of the following:

- Understanding the current managed care environment
- Marketing yourself and your practice to maximize your attractiveness to managed care
- Getting accepted onto managed care panels
- Building a relationship with a managed care organization that generates referrals to your practice
- Reducing liability to avoid issues of potential fraud or abuse
- Getting approvals for your services and avoiding denials of services or payment
- Winning appeals when your services are denied
- Getting paid quickly
- Generating referrals from managed care
- Using the managed care system to generate your own referrals
- Understanding the future directions and opportunities that exist within managed care

As you are probably aware, the managed care environment can be rather complex. Having a basic understanding of how it works and how to communicate with managed care can easily be the difference between getting onto a managed care panel or getting rejected, getting your services approved or denied, completing your paperwork quickly and efficiently or having to rewrite and resubmit it, getting paid quickly or getting paid late or not at all, and generating many new referrals or generating no referrals at all. Throughout this book, you will learn what managed care organizations are looking for from mental health providers and how to give it to them in language they will listen to. You will also learn strategies for thriving within the managed care environment, strategies designed to help you to increase the number of new referrals to your practice in order to generate greater income.

Key Terms

Throughout this book, various managed care terms are used. Therefore, prior to proceeding any further it is important that a few key terms be defined. The term managed care can be applied to many different organizations, including, but not limited to, the health maintenance organization (HMO), preferred provider organization (PPO), and managed behavioral health care organization (MBHO). Generally speaking, an HMO is an organization that contracts with specific medical groups to provide health services to the members of a health plan for a pre paid per-member fee that is paid to individual providers to cover health care services for the members of that health plan (Krieg, 1997). In a PPO, a network of preferred providers is established to provide health care services to the members of the health plan at a reduced fee for the services (Krieg, 1997). MBHO is the term given to the management of behavioral health care that is carved out of the health care plan (regardless of health plan type) to be managed by another agency. The MBHO may be a subsidiary of the health plan or may be an independent company. In either case, the MBHO manages the behavioral health benefits for the health plan.

HMOs, PPOs, and MBHOs are but a few of the possible agencies that can be considered managed care. For the purpose of parsimony, unless otherwise indicated, any organization in which you as a provider can contract to provide mental health services for a fixed reimbursement rate is referred to as a managed care organization (MCO). Similarly, the term *provider* is used to represent any person who provides mental health services. This may include psychiatrists, psychologists, social workers, nurses, marriage and family counselors, and other master's-level therapists. A person covered by an MCO who is treated by a provider can be referred to in different ways. From the perspective of an MCO, this person is generally referred to as a member or a patient. From a mental health provider's perspective, it is generally preferable to refer to this person as a client. However, because this book deals with working within the managed care environment, the terms *member* and *patient* are used, as these are most common within the context of managed care. The term *member* refers to the fact that the person you are treating is a member of the MCO; that is, he or she has health coverage through the MCO. The term *patient* is used in managed care to refer to a member who is being treated for a medical condition. Since the medical model is used to conceptualize psychiatric conditions, *patient* has remained even though most providers would probably prefer to use *client.*

Before beginning the process of looking to become a provider for managed care organizations, it is important to have some background on the current environment of managed care into which you will be entering. Understanding this context is an important and frequently overlooked component of being able to effectively communicate with managed care.

Current Managed Care Context

Behavioral health managed care is a multibillion dollar industry. The leading managed care companies are a mixture of publicly traded companies, privately held companies, and subsidiaries of publicly traded health care companies with mandates for profitability, market share, stock performance, and long-term viability. While the largest MCOs are national, most of them dominate market share in a particular region of the United States. These large, national companies typically have regional care management and provider relations departments who work with local providers and members. You should be aware, however, that in these MCOs, *local* may cover the entire eastern or southern United States, which may not appear very local from your perspective as a provider.

As a provider endeavoring to work within the managed care environment, there are a few current trends that you should be aware of, including the consolidation of health plans, a shift toward bringing behavioral health operations in-house, and the increased influence of outside, evaluative agencies.

Consolidation of Health Plans

Recent years have seen the consolidation of health plans, with many large for-profit health plans buying other relatively smaller health plans. For example, in 2005 United Health announced that it had acquired Pacificare, and WellPoint announced its acquisition of WellChoice. The result of this trend is that there are fewer and fewer MCOs with larger and larger memberships. In fact, an enrollment analysis released in 2004 reported that the top 25 MCOs covered almost 150 million lives while remaining MCOs covered just over 50 million lives (AIS Market Data, 2004). Enrollment in these large plans may also be growing quickly, with the increased enrollment of Medicare and Medicaid members in MCOs (Shlian & Shlian, 1995). With the mergers and acquisitions that have occurred since this analysis was released, the disparity between the few very large MCOs and the smaller ones is sure to be even greater.

While there may be numerous positive and negative complex social repercussions of this health care consolidation trend, there are a few results that may impact you as a provider. With fewer MCOs maintaining greater percentages of the total market, these MCOs will be able to better spread the risk and achieve economies of scale to help lower administrative costs and manage overall medical costs (Shlian & Shlian, 1995). Along with the ability to lower costs, having greater market share gives these large MCOs greater influence when negotiating with providers. While that may not necessarily be good news for providers financially, increased consolidation should mean greater uniformity among MCOs and a reduction in the different types of paperwork that you as a provider will need to be familiar with when working with managed care.

With the rapid acquisitions and consolidation in the industry has come increased competition among the remaining MCOs. With this competition, the industry has seen rapid turnover of enrollees as employers shift coverage to the least costly plan. As a result, MCOs may be less motivated to provide prevention-based interventions that pay off in the future, preferring to focus on shorter-term outcomes. You as a provider should realize that a patient you see today who is covered by a particular MCO may not be covered by that same MCO when you see him or her the following week. You may also be more likely to capture an MCO's attention when addressing short-term as opposed to long-term goals.

Carve-Outs Versus In-House

Mental health benefits are managed with arrangements known as *carve-outs* or *in-house*. In the carve-out arrangement, a managed care plan contracts with a separate organization to provide mental health care for its members (White, 1997). The plan's physicians refer patients with mental health diagnoses to the carve-out company, which manages the treatment and benefits. The carve-out company typically gets paid a per-member per-month fee for each member. If the carve-out company can manage the care for less than the amount received from the MCO, they make a profit. Thus, carve-out companies must work hard to limit the costs associated with mental health service delivery. This arrangement proliferated quickly in the 1990s as MCOs believed that companies specializing in managing mental health benefits could provide the greatest overall savings for the MCO.

Under the in-house arrangement, the MCO itself, not another company, manages the mental health delivery system just as it would its medical delivery system. Currently a significantly greater number of members are managed by carve-out than by in-house arrangements. However, there is a trend toward MCOs bringing their mental health benefits in-house (Duck, 2005; Managed Care Weekly, 2005; White, 1997). For example, Aetna used Magellan as a carve-out to manage its behavioral health units until Aetna, Magellan's largest client, switched from the carve-out arrangement to an in-house arrangement. As of January 1, 2006, Aetna has its own behavioral health unit (Managed Care Weekly, 2005). It is expected that many other MCOs, including WellPoint, will follow suit, reports Morgan Stanley analyst Carl McDonald (Managed Care Weekly, 2005).

As a mental health provider, it is helpful to be aware of whether the MCO you are working with manages mental health benefits in-house or uses a carve-out organization. In a carve-out arrangement, mental health services are kept completely separate from medical services, and patients may often access mental health treatment without the knowledge of the primary care physician, often resulting in a lack of communication between providers (White, 1997). The carve-out organization is under pressure to keep mental health treatment costs low in order to make the largest possible profit. In some cases, medication used for mental health conditions is considered part of the medical benefit and not a mental health cost. Thus, there can even be subtle pressure on the provider to utilize medication over psychotherapy, as medication costs are not factored into the carve-out arrangement.

Increased Influence of Outside Evaluative Agencies

Recent years have seen an increased role and importance of outside evaluative agencies. As you are well aware, the managed care business is highly competitive. MCOs need to attract new members. In particular, MCOs are looking to attract employer groups that purchase health insurance for their employees. These employer groups have a choice of different MCOs and look to purchase health coverage from the MCO that best fits the needs of the organization and its employees. Thus, these employer groups are looking for MCOs that can provide the highest quality health care at the most reasonable cost. In the past, employer groups looking to purchase coverage for employees could compare MCOs based on price but could not easily compare them based on quality. Today, there are agencies dedicated to evaluating the quality of the health care provided by MCOs. The results of these evaluations are then made publicly available to allow for comparisons between MCOs in terms of quality.

The most important and well-known evaluative agency operating within the managed care environment, the National Committee for Quality Assurance (more commonly referred to as NCQA), was created in 1991 and has grown in influence very quickly. In fact, more than half of the HMOs in the nation, covering three quarters of all enrollees, have been reviewed by NCQA (2005a). NCQA is an independent, 501(c)(3) nonprofit organization whose mission is to improve health care quality. According to its Web site, NCQA's vision is to transform health care quality through measurement, transparency, and accountability (NCQA, 2005a). NCQA lists as part of its core values a commitment to provide information that empowers people to make informed decisions about health care. NCQA does this by generating useful, understandable information about health care quality to inform consumer and employer choice (NCQA, 2005a).

MCOs voluntarily apply for NCQA accreditation. The application process is financially costly and involves a rigorous survey that is used to determine whether certain standards designed to evaluate the quality of the MCO's clinical and administrative system are met. That plans are willing to pay to be evaluated by NCQA and undergo this rigorous survey shows you just how important NCQA accreditation has become in the managed care environment. During the survey, the Health Plan Employer Data and Information Set (commonly referred to as HEDIS) is used to measure an MCO's performance on important dimensions of care and service (NCQA, 2005b). All together, HEDIS contains more than 60 different measures focusing on all important aspects of health care (NCQA, 2005), with several of these measures applying directly to the delivery of mental health care.

The growth of NCQA has created great opportunities for mental health providers who understand the HEDIS measures. MCOs need to demonstrate success on these quality measures and will highly value providers who can demonstrate such success, yet few mental health providers working with managed care even know what these measures are. Understanding the measures and how to succeed on them will help you to get services approved quickly and can help increase referrals from the MCO to your practice. Understanding these measures will also help you to put into a meaningful context many of the demands placed on you as a provider by MCOs that may at first seem rather arbitrary. Throughout this book, these measures are explained along with strategies for achieving success in order to grow your practice through managed care.

While NCQA is not the only evaluative agency working with managed care, it is the most commonly used and most highly visible in the health care community. There are, however, other organizations that serve a similar function. For example, the National Business Coalition on Health represents the interests of several large employer groups. These types of organizations develop quality measures similar to NCQA (and even use many of the same measures) and survey MCOs. The results are used by the employer groups to compare MCOs on different quality measures. Organizations such as the National Business Group on Health are used by large companies such as IBM, General Motors, and Marriott to help in selecting health coverage for the millions of employees, retirees, and their families for which the employer groups provide health care. The National Business Group on Health has been particularly beneficial for mental health providers as they strive to protect the mental health needs of consumers and advocate for parity between mental health and medical health care coverage and greater integration between mental health and medical providers. Other organizations that are not tied to employer groups also set standards to which many MCOs need to adhere. One example includes the Utilization Review Accreditation Commission (URAC), whose mission is to promote continuous improvement in the quality and efficiency of heath care management through the process of accreditation and education (URAC, 2005). Another example is the Joint Commission on Accreditation of Healthcare Organizations (JCAHO, pronounced "jay-co"). JCAHO, a nonprofit organization, evaluates and accredits more than 15,000 health care organizations and programs in the United States (JCAHO, 2005). Because NCQA has the greatest penetration in managed care, its measures receive the greatest attention in this book. You should be aware, however, that other measures exist, and whenever an MCO informs you of any quality measures that are being used, you should give attaining success on that measure a high priority.

Now that you have a brief overview of the current managed care environment, it is important to determine if working with managed care is right for you, as working with managed care has both positive and negative aspects.

The Cons of Working With Managed Care

There are several commonly identified disadvantages to working with managed care: low reimbursement, burdensome paperwork, denials of care, and sometimes slow rate of referrals.

Reimbursement

The amount of money MCOs reimburse for services has been cited as a drawback of working with managed care (Psychotherapy Finances, 2000). A *Psychotherapy Finances* survey conducted in 2000 found that responders reported on average that MCOs were reimbursing for individual therapy at a median rate of $95 for psychiatrists, $70 for psychologists, and $60 for social workers, professional counselors, and marriage and family therapists. To some these rates may seem low; to others they may seem fair. Ultimately, it is up to the provider to determine whether the reimbursement offered by an MCO is acceptable or not. While the reimbursement may not be as high as providers would like, for most providers it is difficult to find potential patients that can self-pay at these rates. Providers who are able to find patients able to self-pay these rates are likely to be treating only financially well-off people. For many providers, no longer being able to help patients from lower and middle socioeconomic backgrounds is a major drawback. Thus one of the benefits of working with managed care is being able to work with a very diverse clientele.

Another commonly cited drawback of working with managed care is delays in receiving payment for your services. No matter what MCO you work with, there will be a delay between your delivery of service and your reimbursement from the MCO due to the time necessary to process your claim. This becomes a significant issue for most providers when claims have to be resubmitted because they were not completed properly, resulting in further delays in reimbursement. Fortunately, this book provides you with the strategies necessary to ensure that your claims are submitted correctly so that you will receive payment as soon as possible.

Paperwork

Another common criticism of working with managed care is the added burden of additional paperwork (Appleby, 1997; Spicer, 1998). It is true that a provider working with managed care will have to complete more paperwork and spend more time on paperwork than a provider treating strictly self-pay patients. This additional paperwork tends to become a significant obstacle for providers who do not understand exactly what MCOs are looking for when completing the paper-work, resulting in unnecessary denial of services, delays in payment, or a return of submitted paperwork to be corrected or revised by the provider. While paper-work will probably always be associated with managed care, this book provides strategies for reducing the time spent on paperwork by explaining just what MCOs are looking for and how to give it to them.

Denials of Care

Another potential con associated with managed care is the potential for an MCO to refuse to pay for services that you and your patient feel are necessary. It is easy to understand how this could prove quite frustrating for providers working with managed care. Many providers fail to get services approved because they fail to present their case in a manner most likely to obtain approval from an MCOs or they fail to properly utilize their rights to appeal an MCO's decision. This book ex-plains how MCOs decide whether or not to approve services and provides strate-gies for greatly improving your chances of obtaining authorizations from MCOs, as well as successfully appealing MCO denial decisions.

Rate of Referrals

Upon joining the network of an MCO, some providers expect to receive an immediate deluge of new referrals. In some cases this may occur, but typically it does not. More commonly the rate of referral from the MCO is much slower. Of course, many factors, including the number of MCO members in need of services in your area, and the number of other providers available in your area will affect the rate of referrals you receive. That is why, if you are looking to build your practice, you should look at joining with an MCO as the first step and not a final goal. In order to build your practice while working in managed care, this book provides you with practical strategies for increasing the number of referrals you receive from the MCO and teaches you how to use the MCO's system to generate your own referrals.

The Pros of Working With Managed Care

While payment rates and delays, paperwork, denials of care, and low rates of referral can create drawbacks to working with managed care, particularly for providers who are unaware of the practical strategies presented in this book, working with managed care does offer several advantages to providers. These advantages include a wide range of services, and linkages and integration.

Wide Range of Services

The Center for Mental Health Services (CMHS) has cited several policies for managed care systems. CMHS has stated that managed care systems should ensure that direct services include a continuum of care consisting of, but not limited to, a comprehensive array of flexible community living supports including prevention, treatment, rehabilitation, support, psychiatric rehabilitation, intensive case management, residential treatment, crisis services, and self-help services (CMHS, 2005). Most MCOs also provide access to partial hospital programs, holding beds, respite care, shelters, emergency foster care, home-based assessment, and home care (Feldman & Finguerra, 2001). This wide range of service means that treatment options are not limited to simply outpatient treatment or hospitalization. Thus, managed care offers many different levels of care that can be utilized by your patient as needed in addition to the care you are providing. One service typically offered by MCOs that is of great help to most outpatient mental health providers is the availability of an emergency clinician during working hours and some combination of an on-call clinician and a crisis center after hours (Maltsberger, 2001). This system can facilitate access to a skilled clinician for a member at times when you are not available.

Linkages and Integration

Good managed care systems are well organized and coordinated; all levels of care are accessible; case management is used to ensure continuity of care; and medical and mental health care complement each other (Maltsberger, 2001). The organization and coordination of services central to most MCOs helps link members to appropriate services as soon as they become needed. For example, MCOs have been able to significantly increase the percentage of members discharged from the hospital for a psychiatric condition who then initiate outpatient mental health treatment (Cuffel, Held, & Goldman, 2002; Nelson, Maruish, & Axler, 2000; Reich, Jaramillo, Kaplan, Arciniega, & Kolbasovsky, 2003). In this way, most MCOs are motivated to promote the appropriate use of services, particularly outpatient services, for their members in need. As a result, you as a provider may be the recipient of referrals from an MCO and members are more likely to get the mental health services they need.

As a mental health provider working with managed care, you are also linked with a vast network of medical and mental health providers. The MCO also not only supports you by offering additional specialists for collaboration or concurrent treatment, it also facilitates communication between you and other providers through standards for care that it creates. Therefore, if you are treating someone for panic disorder and want to rule out an underlying thyroid condition as a possible contributor, you can very easily, with the member's consent, speak with the member's primary care physician or speak to other physicians on a variety of other medically related questions. Similarly, if you are treating depression and uncover an underlying substance abuse condition requiring specialty treatment, your MCO can help facilitate entrance into a high-quality substance abuse treatment program.

As a provider working in managed care, you are also more likely to be able to access information about your patient's past treatment. A managed system of care possesses an efficient system of records and promotes efficient sharing of communication between treatment providers (Feldman & Finguerra, 2001). MCOs also tend to limit the number of facilities a member uses while also ensuring that the facilities share an appreciation of the importance of communication and continuity of care. As a provider working alone, obtaining past records can be difficult, but when working with managed care you have a system already set up to assist you in getting the information you need to provide the highest possible quality of care.

Summary Tips

- Pay attention to the consolidation of MCOs in your area.
- Prior to joining an MCO's network, find out if the mental health benefits are managed in-house or by a carve-out company.
- Prior to joining an MCO, try to find out which outside evaluative agencies will be surveying the MCO (e.g., NCQA).
- Weigh the pros and cons of working with managed care to make sure that the managed care environment is a good fit for you and your practice.

Conclusion

For mental health providers, working with managed care offers many exciting opportunities. In the current environment, providers who understand the inner workings of managed care can develop a lucrative and rewarding relationship with managed care. As you read through this book, you will learn how to go about joining managed care. You will also learn strategies for growing your practice with managed care as well as how to reduce or avoid dealing with some of the traditionally less attractive aspects of managed care. By understanding just what MCOs are looking for in providers and in provider communication, you will be prepared to give them exactly what they want so that they can give you what you want—quicker payments, authorizations for services, referrals, and less time dedicated to paperwork.

Once you decide that you as a mental health provider want to enter the world of managed care, the first step is to learn how to market yourself and your practice to be attractive to managed care.

CHAPTER TWO

How to Market Yourself and Your Practice to Managed Care Organizations

Due to the current competitive market in which they operate, MCOs must look to carefully manage costs. One way to accomplish this is to limit the number of providers contracted to provide mental health services to the MCO's members. Therefore, to be successful in marketing yourself and your practice to MCOs, you will need to understand what they are looking for in potential providers and practices. This chapter takes you through the process of making your practice as appealing as possible to MCOs before you begin the actual application and credentialing process. Keep in mind that all MCOs are not the same and that each will have slightly different desired practice characteristics. This chapter presents a general discussion of the office and practice characteristics that MCOs find attractive so that you may model your practice after these criteria as much as possible. In addition to discussing what MCOs are looking for in you as a provider, this chapter also discusses what you should look for in an MCO.

Office Qualities Attractive to Managed Care

When contracting with providers to deliver mental health care for an MCO's members, there are certain qualities that most MCOs will look for. One reason that many MCOs look for similar qualities in providers is not only because these qualities are associated with successful outcomes but because many of them are required by the

NCQA. For example, Pacificare Behavioral Health's (2001b) provider manual lists office and practice requirements, under the heading of "Pacificare Behavioral Health and NCQA Requirements." Knowing the office qualities that are attractive to MCOs should help you shape your practice to meet these needs and to demonstrate to MCOs that your practice incorporates most, if not all, of the qualities they would like to see or require. Generally speaking, office qualities attractive to managed care fall into three main categories: office environment, office safety, and medical record storage.

Office Environment

When an MCO member comes to see you for treatment, you as a provider and your office become a representative of that MCO. It should come as no surprise then that the MCO has a vested interest in being well represented. Therefore, MCOs want to make sure that their members are treated in an environment that is highly professional and clean. Below are typical questions about your practice that an MCO may want to answer when visiting and evaluating your office.

Professionalism
- Is each room equipped with adequate light?
- Does each office contain adequate space?
- Is there a waiting area?
- Does the waiting area contain adequate space?
- Is a restroom available to patients?
- Do visible signs clearly identify your office?
- Does your office space meet the requirements of the Americans with Disabilities Act (U.S. Department of Justice, 2006)?
- Is parking space adequate?
- Is smoking prohibited in your office and waiting room?
- Is soundproofing adequate to protect confidentiality?
- Is your office located in a business, professional, or commercial zone?

Cleanliness
- Does the office appear clean and uncluttered?
- Are the bathrooms kept clean?
- Is there a routine schedule for cleaning?
- Is the exterior of the building clean and adequately maintained?

The more affirmative responses you can give to these questions, the more attractive your practice will be to most MCOs. If you are currently looking to rent office space, be sure to consider these questions before signing a rental agreement. Be sure to consider not only the inside of your office space but the outside of the building as well. Keep in mind that if you become a provider for an MCO, you may be referred members with medical problems or physical disabilities. Therefore every effort should be made to ensure that people with disabilities will be able to access your office.

A common question many providers have is whether or not they will be able to work with managed care patients if they work out of a home office. While there is no yes-or-no answer to this question that will apply to all MCOs, generally speaking, home offices are less attractive to MCOs. That being said, some MCOs will allow you to become a provider and to see their members in a home office, though usually special waivers are required and you will probably need to demonstrate that your office meets all of the criteria listed above. This of course can be difficult to do, as many MCOs, such as Pacificare Behavioral Health (2001b) will want a separate entrance for patients, a waiting area (which should be separate from the living area), and sometimes even a location in a business, professional, or commercial zone. Additional requirements, which are also listed in MHN's (2005) *Practitioner Manual*, include that your office must only be used for business, it may not be used as part of the living area, and it must have a separate phone line that is not accessible to other household residents. Because there are typically many rules for having a home-based office when working with managed care, you should use the rules presented here as a guide and contact any specific MCO you are considering working with to find out all of their specific rules about home-based practices. While having a home-based practice does not preclude you from working with managed care, it can make it much more challenging.

Office Safety

In addition to a professional-looking and clean office, MCOs will expect that your office provide a safe setting for its members. You should take special care to ensure that your office is safe and that care has been taken to demonstrate your commitment to safety. Below is a list of questions regarding office safety an MCO might have about your office:

- Are smoke detectors and fire extinguishers present?
- Are exits clearly marked?

- Is there an emergency evacuation plan?
- Is the area surrounding your office safe, particularly when exiting at night?
- Are emergency phone numbers posted and easily available to staff?
- Are medications protected from public access?
- Are medications securely stored and double locked?

Most of these questions may seem obvious, yet many practices do not take the time to ensure that the answer to each of the questions would be yes in the eyes of an MCO. Regardless of whether or not you are working with an MCO, it is a very good idea to make sure you have plans and preparations already in place in case of an emergency. You should also be sure that all medications (if any are present) are safely locked and stored away. You should also pay close attention to the area around your office. Make sure that the exterior of your office is well lit and safe at night. If safety from crime is an issue, you may need to consider looking for new office space. Not only should your office be reasonably safe from crime, it should be free of other hazards such as large cracks in the concrete, missing steps, and uneven pavement. When judging your office space, try to look at it through the eyes of an MCO that needs to ensure the health and safety of all of its members, including those with the greatest physical limitations.

Medical Record Storage

Proper medical record storage is a critical part of ensuring confidentiality. An MCO wants to be sure that each one of its providers properly protects the confidentiality of its members' medical records. Each MCO should have written policies and procedures in the area of medical record storage and protection of confidentiality. These policies will typically be in line with both federal and state confidentiality regulations and applicable standards set by the NCQA. For example, Pacificare Behavioral Health (2001b) states that providers are required to maintain the confidentiality of all patient health information and other personal information about members. Providers must implement safeguards to ensure confidentiality. Medical records should be stored in such a manner that only the practitioners involved in the member's care, claims processing staff, utilization management and care management staff, quality improvement staff, and other authorized persons shall have access to it (Pacificare Behavioral Health, 2001b). As a provider, it is your responsibility to ensure that all medical records are protected and that only appropriate persons have access to them. Keep in mind that if you are using electronic medical records, each staff member or practitioner in the practice should have a unique password to ensure that only authorized persons have access to records. It is a good idea to have each office staff member sign a confidentiality agreement, which should be kept on file in your office. Given the importance of confidentiality, it should come as no surprise that MCOs expect providers to demonstrate commitment to proper storage of records and will include measures of this in most if not all audits. As you will see in later chapters, audits can occur at any time. Therefore, when reviewing your practice as you prepare to join an MCO network, consider the following questions:

- Are all medical records filed away or are some left out?
- Are medical records filed securely?
- Are files locked?
- Who has access to the files? Do any unauthorized personnel have access to the files?
- Are your records easily retrievable?
- Are your records clearly organized?
- Are your records bound?
- Do your records contain a confidentiality policy demonstrating that you have discussed issues of confidentiality with your patients?

Practice Qualities Attractive to Managed Care

In addition to physical office qualities that are attractive to managed care, MCOs will also look for certain practice qualities that make a provider and his or her practice more appealing. Important practice qualities attractive to managed care include access to care, general service standards, and clinician skills.

Access to Care

MCOs want to be sure that their members are able to get an appointment for treatment in a timely manner. This is not only to promote adequate treatment of behavioral health conditions but to promote a satisfied membership. MCOs will expect their providers to meet certain criteria for timeliness.

Access standards are monitored carefully throughout the managed care industry. Different MCOs may have different access standards but, generally speaking, most will adopt the criteria developed by NCQA. Table 2.1 presents the standard for each of the commonly reported access types. In order to provide timely access and to monitor your practice's access, you first need to know how to classify your

TABLE 2.1. **Standards for Access to Care**

Access Type	Standard
Life-threatening emergency	Seen immediately
Non-life-threatening emergency	Seen within 6 hours
Urgent care	Seen within 48 hours
Routine care	Seen within 10 days

appointments into the categories in Table 2.1. This can be somewhat confusing, particularly when it comes to distinguishing between a life-threatening and non-life-threatening emergency. Not all MCOs will clearly differentiate definitions for each type of appointment classification, so when working with an MCO it is a good idea to ask for clarification, especially if the topic is not covered adequately in the MCO's provider manual (described in Chapter 4). One organization that has taken the time to define each type of appointment in its provider manual is APS Healthcare (2003):

- Life-threatening emergency—A situation in which a member has made a suicide attempt or is in immediate danger of making a suicide attempt.
- Non-life-threatening emergency—A situation in which the member is markedly distressed and there is a strong potential for rapid decompensation.
- Urgent Care—A situation in which a member's condition could be anticipated to deteriorate to the point of being at risk of harm to self or others if not evaluated or treated within 48 hours.
- Routine Care—An appointment is to be offered within 10 business days of the initial referral for routine care.

Keep in mind that while these standards and their definitions are generally accepted throughout managed care, certain MCOs may adopt slightly different and more stringent standards or definitions. In some cases, national MCOs may even have different standards in different areas. For example, APS Healthcare (2003) has adopted the above criteria but reports in its provider manual that New York State providers are expected to see urgent care appointment within 24 hours as opposed to 48 hours and routine care appointments within 7 days as opposed to 10 days. Of course, the faster you are able to see members referred to you, the more attractive you and your practice will be to managed care. While 10 days may seem like plenty of time in which to schedule a routine appointment, many MCOs view 10 days as an absolute maximum time frame. For example, Pacificare Behavioral Health's (2001b) provider manual states that a routine appointment should be offered within 5 business days of the referral and that the provider should ensure that the member will be seen within 10 business days.

You should also be aware that some MCOs, such as Magellan Behavioral Health (2004), ask members to inform them whenever a provider fails to offer a routine appointment within 10 days. While the emphasis on strict access standards may feel like an unnecessary burden at times to providers, MCOs must monitor performance on these access standards in order to comply with NCQA standards. In fact, most MCOs have to report the performance of their providers on a semi-annual basis. You should also keep in mind that your patient's definition of an emergency appointment may not be the same as the MCO's definition, such as when an evaluation is needed for a child to return to school or an adult to return to work. Whenever possible, you should do your best to meet the patient's needs, as patient satisfaction is also very important to MCOs.

SPOTLIGHT ON

Providing Timely Access

A psychiatrist was on the panel of an MCO for over 4 months without receiving a single referral from the MCO. Then one Friday, she received a call in the late afternoon from the MCO's case management department informing her that they needed an appointment for a man who was just discharged from the hospital after a 7-day admission due to a manic episode. The psychiatrist was already booked for the rest of the day and did not have an available appointment until the following Friday morning. She notified the MCO of this and then let the MCO know that she considers post-psychiatric hospital discharge appointments to be of the highest priority, and agreed to stay at her office late and see the MCO's member at the end of the day after all of her other appointments. After seeing this member, the psychiatrist noted that she started to get referrals from the MCO on a fairly regular basis, particularly members that were recently discharged from the hospital. The lesson here is that providing timely access, particularly for urgent and emergency appointments, is one of the best ways to gain the attention and favor of an MCO.

Generally speaking, from a managed care perspective, group practices tend to offer a greater potential for quicker access, greater coverage, and more available time slots for MCO members. Many MCOs therefore may have a preference for providers working in a group practice as opposed to practicing on their own. That is not to say that a provider practicing alone cannot work with managed care, only that some MCOs may give preference to providers working in group practices. Therefore, joining a group practice, particularly one with experience working with managed care, may be helpful for someone looking to get started working in the managed care environment.

SPOTLIGHT ON

Joining a Group Practice

A psychologist with 2 years of experience since becoming licensed started a private practice. To build his practice, he attempted to join the networks of two MCOs in his area but was unsuccessful. He then joined a group practice, reapplied several months later, and was accepted into one of the networks. Approximately 1 year later, he left the group practice to restart his individual practice, maintaining his status as a credentialed provider for the MCO, and continued to receive referrals as an independent practitioner. While joining a group is certainly no guarantee of getting into MCO networks, in many cases it can make it somewhat easier.

General Service Standards

In addition to seeing referrals without a long waiting period, MCOs expect your practice to provide a certain level of service to their members. While each MCO may have slightly different expectations, most will expect that their members' routine phone calls will be returned by the next business day, urgent phone calls will be returned within one hour, and any type of emergency phone call will be returned immediately. You should also be sure to have instructions detailing what members should do in an emergency if they get your answering machine or service. For example, your message might say, "If this is an emergency, dial zero for the operator, who will connect you to me immediately" or at the very least, "If this is an emergency, you should hang up and dial 911."

All patients should also be informed about how they can contact you during and after business hours in an urgent or emergency situation. This is particularly important to MCOs, as an MCO member in an urgent or emergency situation who is unable to contact his or her provider in a timely manner is likely to go directly to an emergency room, even when this level of care is not necessary. This may represent unneeded use of limited emergency room resources and an increased expenditure to the MCO that could easily have been avoided if the member was able to reach the provider. This is of particular concern to MCOs, as studies have demonstrated the overuse of the emergency room for psychiatric services (Claasen et al., 2000; Dhossche & Ghani, 1998; Marchesi et al., 2004; Zdanowicz, Janne, Gillet, Reynaert, & Vause, 1996).

Most MCOs will prefer practices in which at least one staff member is available for patient intake during business hours. Many MCOs also like providers to utilize patient educational materials and to coordinate efforts with primary care physicians (PCPs). Providers who have a system for sending reports to their patients' PCPs are going to be attractive to MCOs, as most MCOs believe in the importance of coordination between providers, particularly when a patient was referred by the PCP, has comorbid medical conditions, has comorbid substance abuse issues, or is on psychiatric medication. Many MCOs also like to see that a list of patients' rights and responsibilities is either handed out or displayed in your office or waiting area.

Finally, and perhaps unsurprisingly, many MCOs, such as APS Healthcare (2003) and Pacificare Behavioral (2001b), will state a preference for providers, particularly therapists, to demonstrate adherence to time-limited therapy. You should keep in mind that appropriateness of care is very important to MCOs (Hiatt & Hargrave, 1995). This does not mean that every patient can only be seen for a short period of time. It does mean that the amount of time you see someone should be influenced by a number of factors including diagnosis, symptom severity, and risk of decompensation if treatment is not provided. For example, an MCO is likely to frown upon a provider who has treated a patient weekly for 2 years for an adjustment disorder with little demonstrated progress. That same MCO is likely to look favorably upon a provider who has worked with a patient with schizophrenia or bipolar disorder for the same time period while working toward maintaining medication adherence and avoiding psychiatric hospitalizations and emergency room visits.

Clinician Skills

MCOs prefer to work with practices that employ highly skilled providers. Obviously, providers with a demonstrated record of ethical behavior who deliver evidence-supported treatment to patients while also taking into consideration the customer service aspect of providing care are going to be more attractive to MCOs. In response to managed care's policies calling for cost containment, attention to outcomes, practice audits, and treatment guidelines, several additional clinician skills attractive to managed care have been identified: population-oriented practice management and development, command of a broad repertoire of methodologies, and ethical analysis (Sabin, 1991).

Because MCOs are in the business of managing an entire population of members they tend to think in terms of populations, whereas providers tend to be more concerned with the individuals with whom they are working. A provider who thinks in terms of populations is likely to balance time spent on each member with maintaining availability for other potential members. By thinking in terms of populations, you will have a better idea of an MCO's thought processes. A broad repertoire of methodologies is important because an MCO covers a wide variety of people and behavioral health conditions. Any provider working within managed care is going to need to be able to handle a very diverse clientele. In addition, the federal government now requires state Medicaid programs to offer culturally competent services, although little is known about how mandates related to cultural competency are monitored or enforced (Stork, Scholle, Greeno, Copeland, & Kelleher, 2001). Nevertheless, more and more MCOs are stating a preference for providers who demonstrate culturally sensitive work or have experience working with patients from different cultural backgrounds.

Up to this point, this chapter has detailed many of the characteristics most MCOs find attractive in potential behavioral health providers. As a provider looking to build a practice within the managed care environment, you should try to adopt as many of these characteristics in your practice as possible. However, you should also consider what qualities are attractive to *you* in an MCO.

Choosing the Right MCO for You

Some providers looking to join with MCOs simply identify as many MCOs in their area as possible and submit applications to join all of their networks without taking the time to learn about the organizations at all. While it is true that there is a great deal of similarity between MCOs in terms of what they request require of providers, particularly as many MCOs need to report results on many of the same measures to NCQA or other organizations, MCOs will still differ on several issues that will be important to you as a provider. For example, some MCOs are requesting more outcome-based assessments. Some MCOs will be faster than others in terms of processing claims. Some MCOs will have providers relations departments that are more helpful than others and some will generate more referrals to their providers than others. MCOs are also likely to differ in the type of provider specialties they are looking for and the number of covered lives they manage. For example, an MCO that services a high volume of diverse Medicaid members may place a higher value on your experience treating a very culturally diverse population. Similarly, an MCO that services a high volume of Medicare members will be likely to place a high value on your experience working with the elderly and the ability to discriminate between dementia and pseudodementia. When looking to join with an MCO, you should be careful to consider not only what the MCO wants in its providers, but just how good a match that MCO is for you. Below is a list of questions to help you determine what qualities you should look for in an MCO.

Financial

- How much do I need to get paid per session for the work to be worth my while (remember you need to factor in time for paperwork)?
- Can I get paid for 30-minute sessions as opposed to 50-minute sessions? Am I interested in 30-minute sessions?
- Can I get paid for doing group work? Am I interested in doing group work?
- What is the average wait time between submission of a claim and receipt of payment?
- How important is speed of payment to me?
- Will I receive any payment if an MCO member does not show up for a scheduled appointment?
- Can I contract with a member directly to be reimbursed a fee in an appointment is broken without notice?
- How is the MCO doing financially as an organization? Do I think it will be around for awhile?

Administrative

- How much paperwork is involved?
- Will I find the paperwork complicated and difficult to complete accurately?
- Can I maintain a level of organization in terms of handling paperwork that is sufficient to handle the MCO's demand for information?

- Does the MCO need outcome assessments integrated into my work? Is that a problem or will I find these measures useful?
- How often does the MCO conduct chart audits? How does it determine who will be audited? How prepared would I be for a chart audit?
- Can I provide the required access for routine, urgent, and emergency appointments?

Services

- How easy or difficult is it to get in touch with someone at the MCO?
- Does the MCO have people available who can answer any questions that come up?
- How satisfied are the MCO's members with the behavioral health services offered by that MCO?
- How satisfied are the MCO's members with the customer service that MCO provides?

Membership

- What type of membership does the MCO have? Am I interested in treating those members?
- Does my clinical expertise match well with the type of members the MCO would be likely to refer?

Influence in Your Area

- How many people in my geographic area are covered by the MCO?
- Can I handle a large influx of new patients? Can I afford not to join the MCO if it has a strong penetration rate in my area?
- Are there rumors of a large national MCO acquiring local MCOs in the area? If so, you may need to join the local MCOs quickly, so that if they are acquired you do not get shut out of the network, especially if the national MCO will cover most of the potential patients in your area.

As you answer these questions, you should have a better understanding of what type of MCO would fit you best. For example, if you are a very organized and detailed provider with a small practice that you are under pressure to grow quickly, an MCO that requires a great deal of paperwork including outcome measures might be fine, but an MCO that is slow in processing claims may create problems for you. On the other hand, a less organized provider with a large practice may not mind delays in getting paid as the practice has other sources of revenue but may have difficulties with an MCO requiring a great deal of paperwork. As you decide what characteristics are most important to you, the next step is to do your market research to find the MCOs in your area that seem to be the best fit for you.

SPOTLIGHT ON

Getting Information on Your Local MCO

In addition to browsing an MCO's Web site and NCQA's Web site, consider accessing any professional organization of which you may be a member, such as the American Psychiatric Association. Some organizations will provide information about MCOs or results from surveys about their members' experience with particular MCOs. A psychologist recently reported using the Web site of a professional organization to identify members with backgrounds dealing with managed care. By contacting a few of these members, she was able to find out that one of the two MCOs she was considering joining had a good reputation among the organization's members, while the other had a very poor reputation. Armed with this information, she was able to focus all of her energies on trying to join the network of the MCO with the good reputation.

The Role of Market Research

Thanks to the internet, today providers have much more information available to them about MCOs than ever before. Once you have figured out which MCO characteristics are most important to you, take the time to visit each organization's Web site. From the Web site you should be able to find out important information such as how the MCO functions, where its providers and members are located, and contact information for staff in the provider relations department. More and more, MCOs are including copies of the forms that are required of their providers as well as frequently asked provider questions with answers. Within a few minutes of browsing an MCO's Web site, you should have a pretty good sense of how it operates and how well that MCO would suit you. For additional questions that have not been answered, consider simply calling the MCO's provider relations department. It is also a good idea to visit the NCQA Web site (www.NCQA.org) to search for any additional information or report cards on that MCO.

As you review the materials on an MCO's Web site, keep in mind the source of that information. It is highly unlikely that any negative information is going to be reported by the MCO on its own site. The best information will come from providers already working with a particular MCO. Therefore, you should take the time find out what MCOs some of your colleagues and friends have worked with. If you know someone who has worked with the MCO, be sure to ask questions like: "How quickly do they handle claims?", "What is the process for requesting additional sessions?", "How much time do you spend with paperwork?" If you can not find anyone who has worked with the MCO, check the MCO's list of providers (often available online) for names and numbers of providers in your area. Then simply call one or two of them, introduce yourself, and ask them your questions. Most providers should be willing to spend a few minutes talking to you as a professional courtesy. After all, they were once trying to join with managed care as well.

SPOTLIGHT ON

Questioning Providers Already in an MCO's Network

When contacting a provider who is already a member of an MCO you are interested in joining, you should ask any questions that are relevant to you and your decision to join that MCO. Below is a list of questions you might consider asking:

- What is the reimbursement rate?
- Have you had difficulties getting reimbursed for your services?
- Is there a great deal of oversight by the MCO?
- Have you had difficulties getting needed services approved?
- Has the MCO referred many members to you?
- How satisfied are you with the MCO?
- Is the MCO staff helpful when you need assistance?

After you have done your market research and identified MCOs that you are interested in joining as a provider, and after you have set up your office and your practice to be attractive to managed care, there is one more step before you are ready to begin the process of applying to join an MCO network: You should find out which MCOs your current caseload of patients belong to. If you are currently seeing patients who are paying you out of pocket but have insurance with mental

---

SPOTLIGHT ON

Getting Credentialed to Treat a Single Member

A boy named Johnny was identified as having behavioral problems, ADHD, and comorbid Tourette's syndrome. Johnny and his family resided in a community with few child psychology specialists, and practically none with a specialty in working with Tourette's syndrome. The MCO provided the family with a child psychiatrist who prescribed medication and referred the child for psychotherapy to address social adjustment and behavioral issues. The psychiatrist referred the child to a local colleague with experience working with Tourette's, who agreed to take on the case even though she was not a part of the provider network of the family's MCO. When the mother discovered that this provider was not in the managed care network, she called the care manager of the MCO and requested that the visits to this child psychologist be covered since her child had a combination of disorders requiring special professional skills. The care manager called the child psychologist directly and arranged for the care to be approved at a mutually agreed-upon fee, which was very close to the psychologist's customary charge.

After dealing with the child psychologist on this difficult case, the care manager sent the child psychologist a credentialing application, requesting that she become a participating provider in the MCO's network. The child psychologist decided to join the network, and because of her special training and expertise was identified as a privileged provider. The child psychologist was the beneficiary of additional referrals in two ways: first, directly from the MCO and second, from the local psychiatrist who was now aware that his colleague was a participating provider with the same managed care organization.

health benefits, you should discuss the prospect of joining their MCO as a provider. Assuming that a patient has no objections to using his or her mental health benefits, you can call that patient's MCO and request to be credentialed to see that MCO's member and to be paid for your services by that MCO. It is unlikely that the MCO will take you on as a full provider at that point, but some will agree to pay you for future services to that particular member without having to go through the formal credentialing process. If you can get such an agreement, your foot is in the door. As you build up a history of delivering quality service, you will be gaining experience with that MCO and should have an even better chance of eventually joining the MCO as a full provider in the future.

Once you have designed your practice and your office to maximize attractiveness, identified MCOs you are interested in joining, and made contact with the MCOs of your current caseload, you are ready for the next, all-important step: getting into managed care networks.

Summary Tips

- Make sure your office looks professional.
- Make sure your office is clean.
- Make sure your office is safe.
- Ensure the confidentiality of your files (whether paper or electronic).
- Have a policy for ensuring you will meet all access standards.
- Make sure you have a policy for how patients should contact you in an urgent or emergency situation (and make sure your patients are aware of the policy).
- Search the internet for information about any MCO you are interested in working with.
- Talk to providers already working with MCOs you are interested in.
- Try to join with MCOs of patients you are currently treating.
- Select MCOs that are a good fit for you.
- Due to the trend of consolidation in managed care, you should strongly consider joining an MCO that dominates the market in your area, as this MCO may soon become even larger, representing an even greater potential source of referrals.

CHAPTER THREE

Getting Into Managed Care Networks

Once you have set up your practice to maximize its attractiveness to managed care you will need to pursue getting into an MCOs network. This chapter describes the process of joining an MCO network by successfully negotiating the credentialing process. The process of requesting and completing an application to join an MCO network is explained, followed by a description of common pitfalls that delay applications and tips for submitting a successful application. Finally, what to expect if your application is accepted and tips for handling a rejection letter are described.

Provider Networks

In order to receive payment to treat an MCO's member, you must first be in that MCO's network of providers. A network or panel consists of all service providers that are approved to provide services to the members of an insurance plan (Krieg, 1997). Each health plan maintains a network of mental health providers that are qualified to deliver high-quality care to its members. The size of an MCO's network is based on the number of providers needed to deliver services to the MCO's members. To ensure quality and control costs, MCOs carefully manage their provider networks. They set provider standards to ensure that all providers meet a minimum standard of education, experience, and licensing.

In addition to establishing standards for providers, MCOs establish standards regarding the total number of providers required to service a geographic area based on membership in that area. While these standards may seem capricious at times to providers, the number of providers in an area is often dictated by standards created by outside evaluative agencies. Because of the high cost of credentialing and managing providers as well as the cost of providing care, most MCOs are careful not to accept additional providers once they feel they have attained the minimum number needed to deliver care to members in a given area. When no more providers are being accepted in a given area, the network is said to be closed. MCOs also manage costs through their contracts with providers in their networks. When a provider signs a contract to provide services to an MCO's members, he or she agrees to the MCO's contracted rate. This contracted rate, which is often lower than the provider's normal rate, allows the MCO to control costs and to better estimate the cost of providing services to its members.

It should come as no surprise that MCOs are looking to achieve a network with a limited number of highly qualified providers that agree to a specific fee schedule and provide services in convenient locations for their members. To fit into this system, any mental health care provider looking to join an MCO's network will need to undergo a rather substantial credentialing process.

Overview of the Credentialing Process

When applying to an MCO's network, you will go through a thorough evaluation of your credentials and experience. The credentialing process ensures that prospective providers meet all of the criteria set forth by the MCO's credentialing committee. In most cases, the MCO's credentialing process also ensures compliance with guidelines set forth by NCQA. While each MCO will have its own specific credentialing process, several steps in the credentialing process are fairly uniform across MCOs.

Step One: Requesting and Submitting an Application

The first step in the credentialing process is to request an application to join the network. Once your application is received, carefully completed with all supporting documentation, and returned to the MCO's provider relations department, it may or may not be reviewed for completeness and then will be forwarded to the credentialing committee, which typically meets once every three months. If a reviewer or a member of the credentialing committee finds that the application is not complete in any way, the application will be returned and will need to be completed and resubmitted. In many cases this means that the credentialing process will have to start over. Even something as small as forgetting to check a particular box can result in a delay of months, which can mean having to wait until the next credentialing committee meeting for your application to be reviewed. Therefore, submitting a correctly completed application is of the utmost importance.

Step Two: The Credentialing Committee Review

Assuming that your application has been fully completed, the application and all supporting documents are reviewed by the MCO's credentialing committee. Typically, all information goes through primary source verification, a process that will likely conform to NCQA standards. The MCO, or an outside organization contracted to perform the primary source verification process, will verify that all information provided in the application is correct. This verification is achieved through communication with a variety of outside agencies, including but not limited to state boards of licensure or certification, the National Practitioner Data Bank (NPDB), state boards of examiners, federations of medical boards, and regional Medicare and Medicaid offices. The MCO is also likely to do a background check to discover any possible criminal record. Because of the depth of the verification process and for ethical reasons, it is critically important to be honest and complete with all information provided in your application to join a network.

You should assume that anything in the public record will become known to the MCO even if it is not asked about in the application. Provider relations staff members of several MCOs have reported many cases of rejecting applicants because information was discovered during the primary source verification process that was not explained or mentioned by the applicant. Most if not all applications will provide an opportunity to explain any past claims against you or other situations that need elaboration. It is highly recommended that rather than hiding information, you take the opportunity to clearly explain any past situations that could potentially negatively impact the status of your application.

The results of the primary source verification and all application materials are reviewed and potentially approved by the credentialing committee. In many MCOs, the credentialing committee will at this time decide to accept or reject an applicant. Some large national MCOs may have an additional step whereby the local division of that MCO must approve of all prospective providers and then forward all information to a national credentialing committee, which must also approve of the applicants.

SPOTLIGHT ON

Primary Source Verification

A psychologist licensed in the states of New York and California was sanctioned by California for failing to provide a comprehensive evaluation in a custody case. The corrective action plan included the psychologist's submission to a 1-year period of supervision in which all evaluations had to be countersigned by the supervisor. Fearing the damage this would do to her business, the psychologist decided to return to New York and continue practicing independently and without supervision. She applied to join the network of an MCO in New York State and submitted all licensing information pertaining to her New York license, omitting any reference to the sanctions imposed on her in California. During primary verification, the MCO discovered the events that occurred in California and the psychologist's application was rejected. The lesson here is that you cannot hide from primary source verification. Instead, take the time to explain any events that could negatively impact your application.

Step Three: The MCO Decision

Given all that is involved in the credentialing process and the infrequency with which most credentialing committees typically meet, it is not surprising that the credentialing process is a slow one. How long it takes will vary by MCO, but almost all will complete the process within 3 to 6 months from the time the application is received to inform you of whether your application to join the network has been accepted or rejected. While MCOs differ in how long they take to notify applicants of a decision, the NCQA guidelines give MCOs 6 months in which to complete the credentialing process. As a result, most plans will complete the process within that time frame. Thus, if your application is submitted and a response is not received within 6 months, it is a good idea to contact the MCO to inquire about the status of the application. Because the credentialing process is lengthy, it is also a good idea to call the MCO 2 weeks after submitting your application to ensure it has been received, as many MCOs will not contact you to verify that it was received. If you do not call to confirm receipt and it gets lost, it may be

6 months before someone discovers the problem. Once you have verified that your application was received, be patient. Written notification of the MCO's decision should occur within 6 months.

While the credentialing process will vary from MCO to MCO, the structure of the credentialing process described above is fairly standard. Therefore, to become part of a network, you will need to start by obtaining an application.

SPOTLIGHT ON

Verifying Receipt of Your Application Materials

A social worker meticulously completed all aspects of the credentialing application and prior to sending in the materials made sure that the MCO was still accepting providers into its network from her area. After not hearing anything back from the MCO in 7 months, she decided to call to find out the status of her application. A provider relations staff member unhappily informed her that they had no record of her application, even though the social worker knew exactly when she had sent the materials and even kept a copy of the postage receipt. The staff member told the social worker that there was nothing he could do but send her a new application. The social worker, eager to join the network, completed a new application and got all of the accompanying materials. This time she called to verify that the materials she sent were received, which they were. Several months later, after the credentialing committee reviewed her application, the social worker received a notice that despite her qualifications her application was denied because the network was closed in her area. It had been closed only 2 months prior to the committee's decision. The lesson here is never to assume that the MCO has received your materials. In fact, assume that they did not.

Requesting an Application

Currently there are two main ways to obtain an application: the Web and the telephone. The Web sites of some MCOs actually allow you to download the application to join the network directly from the Web site. While this is very convenient, as yet the majority of MCOs do not have this option. It is expected, however, that in the future MCO Web sites will become more interactive, with many more MCOs making their applications available online.

If you download applications from the internet, be aware that quite a few MCOs now require you to complete an online request in order to receive an application. This request typically asks you to provide background information in such areas as training, education, licensing, liability insurance, and location. By doing this MCOs, hope to deny requests of providers that do not meet minimum criteria prior to even submitting an application, thus limiting the number of applications that go through the expensive and time-consuming process of credentialing. It is good to review this request to help determine if you will meet the MCO's criteria before investing any further time and effort into preparing an application.

Most Web sites not offering the application online will at least instruct you to call the MCO's provider relations department directly and will provide the contact phone number. If the Web is not being used or the number is not provided, simply look up the main number for the MCO and ask to be transferred to behavioral health provider relations. If calling for an application, you should be sure to verify from the person handling the call that the MCO is currently accepting providers into the network from your area. Questions regarding the MCO's criteria for experience and licensing are also helpful to ensure the application will not be rejected for failing to meet the specified criteria. Once your request is made and your application received, it is helpful to know what to expect.

What to Expect on an Application to Join a Network

Each MCO will have its own specific application to join its network. Each MCO will ask for slightly different information and will have slightly different minimum criteria and standards, so applicants should be prepared to spend a fair amount of time and effort completing each application individually. Generally speaking, MCOs do not prevent or frown upon you joining as many other MCO networks as you like. However, before trying to join every MCO panel in your area, you should keep in mind that the best applications are those which clearly provide the specific information desired by each specific MCO. Thus each application should be tailored for the specific organization to which it will be sent, making the completion of many applications at once quite difficult. While each application will be different, generally speaking there are several areas that you can expect to be present: educational requirements, licensing requirements, experience requirements, and verification of liability insurance. Also, applications will have additional requirements for psychiatrists, may ask for a variety of other supporting documents, and may even include a copy of the provider contract.

SPOTLIGHT ON

Verifying Experience Requirements

A newly licensed psychologist interested in joining a particular MCO's network reviewed information available on the MCO's Web site and found that a minimum of one year of experience was required. He had received his license 6 months previously, prior to which he worked for 12 months as a postdoctoral intern. The psychologist considered himself to have 18 months' experience, but to be sure he called and asked the MCO if all of his work experience counted from the MCO's perspective. He was informed that this MCO required 1 year of experience as a licensed psychologist. As a result, the psychologist did not waste his time rushing to submit an application right away. Instead, he carefully prepared his application over the next several months and submitted it once he had the full 12 months' experience.

Educational Requirements

MCOs will typically require you to possess the highest training applicable to your profession. Therefore, it will be expected that a social worker applying to the network will possess a master's degree in social work, a marriage and family counselor will have a master's degree in marriage and family counseling, a psychologist will possess a doctorate in psychology, a psychiatrist will possess a medical doctor (MD) degree. Some MCOs—not all—will require that a provider's degree be from an accredited college, university, or professional school, and an Education Commission for Foreign Medical Graduates (ECFMG) certificate may be required for physicians completing their training outside of the United States. Because different MCOs will have slightly different educational requirements, it is important to carefully read the application's section on educational requirements. For verification, MCOs may ask for a photocopy of your degree. Also be aware that during the credentialing process the MCO may also contact your college, university, or professional school to verify your degree. Thus, any issues that could result in your former school being less than cooperative should be resolved prior to the submission of your application.

SPOTLIGHT ON

Educational Requirements

A social worker recently applied to join an MCO network. She carefully completed all aspects of the application and made sure that she met all of the necessary educational and other requirements. When she did not get a response from the MCO in over 6 months, she called to find out the reason why she had not heard back. She was informed that her graduate school refused to send proof that she received her master's degree. When she called the school to find out why proof was not sent, she was informed of the school's policy not to comply with such requests unless all fees were paid in full. It turned out that she was issued a parking ticket on campus of which she was unaware and consequently never paid. This one minor oversight caused a 9-month delay in her credentialing.

Licensing Requirements

All MCOs will demand that you are licensed in the state in which you practice. Typically, MCOs expect that you are currently licensed at the highest level with no restrictions. Some MCOs may also specify a particular length of time that a license must be maintained.

Experience Requirements

MCOs will generally also demand that you have a certain amount of experience prior to joining the network. The experience criteria generally range from 2 to 5 years. Some MCOs will begin counting hours or years of experience from the time you obtained your degree, while others will count from the time you became licensed. In general, if you have less than 5 years experience, be sure to find out exactly how much experience is required and how the MCO calculates experience. You should also assume that during the credentialing process the MCO will verify your complete employment history.

Verification of Liability Insurance

It is expected that you maintain liability insurance. Most MCOs will require you to maintain liability coverage of $1 million per occurrence and $3 million aggregate. Some MCOs now require physician providers to maintain $1 million/$3 million but will allow psychologists and social workers to maintain a lower policy of $1 million per occurrence and $1 million aggregate. For liability purposes and to ensure acceptability for a much greater number of MCOs, it is recommended that you maintain at least $1million/$3 million coverage at all times.

Failing to document the proper amount of liability coverage will result in a denial of your application to join a network. Liability insurance, even when the proper amount is documented, is a common obstacle and reason for the denial of many applications. The reason is that, as mentioned previously, the process of credentialing can take up to 6 months. If your submitted liability policy expires during those 6 months, the application can be denied or at a minimum delayed, even if you have since renewed your policy. This is quite common since liability insurance contracts are usually renewed yearly, and credentialing can take up to 6 months. For this reason, it is strongly recommended that when submitting proof of liability insurance, you make sure that your proof of liability coverage will be valid for a minimum of 6 months from the date that your application is received by the MCO. If your coverage will expire during the credentialing process, you should be sure to review your policy prior to termination and immediately send a copy of the renewal notice to the MCO and call to verify that it was received. This seemingly small step prior to submitting an application can save a great deal of difficulty and delay later on in the process.

Additional Requirements for Psychiatrists

There is additional documentation that most MCOs will require of psychiatrists looking to join a network. MCOs will typically ask potential psychiatrists to submit a copy of a valid Controlled Dangerous Substance (CDS) certificate and/or a valid Drug Enforcement Agency (DEA) certificate. As always, you should make sure that these documents will not expire within 6 months of submission. MCOs will generally also require documentation that you have admitting privileges at a hospital. In most if not all cases, having an admitting privilege at more than one hospital is highly desirable to MCOs. Thus, if possible, when looking to join networks, try to obtain admitting privileges at a second (or more) hospital to strengthen your application. If you do have multiple admitting privileges, make this explicit in the application even if the application does not specifically ask about admitting privileges at more than one facility. If you do not have admitting privileges in at least one facility and are still allowed to apply to the network, it is a good idea to include a description of an adequate process for providing emergency care for any patients in need of immediate hospitalization.

It is important to read the application of each MCO carefully as applications differ in what additional physician requirements are present. For example, some MCOs will give preference to psychiatrists who are board certified while others will require psychiatrists to be board certified before they are eligible to join the network. Therefore, one way to strengthen an application is to become board certified, particularly in such specialties as psychiatry or neurology. Psychiatrists specializing in addictions may be particularly appealing to MCOs if they are certified by the American Society of Addiction Medicine (ASAM). Information about becoming certified by ASAM is available on their Web site at www.asam.org.

As mentioned previously, some MCOs will require documentation that accredited residency training has been completed. If you graduated from medical school outside the United States, you may be required to document an ECFMG in order to join the network. Be sure to take the time to carefully read all the additional requirements for psychiatrists. As always, it should be assumed that the MCO will verify that each requirement has been met.

Other Supporting Documents

In addition to documentation of educational, licensing, experience, and liability insurance requirements, most applications to join an MCO's network include requests for several other documents. The most common of these are a curriculum vitae (CV), letters of recommendation, and attestations. Some applications will also include a provider contract.

Curriculum Vitae
Almost all applications will require you to include a CV. The CV should accurately reflect your work history as the MCO is very likely to verify its accuracy. Any gaps in your work history greater than 6 months should be explained. For example, a therapist who worked at a mental health center for 5 years and then left that job after having a baby, and returned to work at a different facility part time 1 year later, should explain this in a letter included with the application materials. This should be done even if the gap occurred several years ago. Some applications will

explicitly state that your CV should be no more than 3 months old and that gaps in work history of greater than 6 months should be explained, while other applications will not. As a general rule, applicants are strongly advised to update their CV just prior to submitting the application and to put a small notation at the end of the CV stating "last updated [date of application submission]" and to include a brief letter explaining any gaps in work history. As a general rule, a CV should include at least a 5-year work history.

Your CV should be a clearly written, accurate portrait of you with no typographical errors. Before submitting your CV, you should review the MCO's application and Web site to gain a better understand of what is highly valued or preferred in providers of that MCO. For example, many MCOs are looking for providers with specialties in the treatment of children and adolescents, geriatric populations, and the chronically mentally ill. If you plan to declare a specialty working with these (or other) populations, be sure to emphasize this type of work experience on your CV. Most MCOs also value previous experience working with managed care. Any previous experience working with managed care should clearly be highlighted in your CV.

Most MCOs will also highly value clinicians with multicultural experience. If you have such experience, be sure to highlight it in your CV. One of the greatest assets you can possess in terms of joining a network is to be fluent in a foreign language. Almost all MCOs will give preference to bilingual clinicians. Detail all foreign language fluencies on the first page of your CV.

In addition to foreign languages, some MCOs prefer their providers to be members of an organization with an ethics code. Therefore, physicians should document membership in the American Medical Association or American Psychiatric Association, psychologists in the American Psychological Association, social workers in the National Association of Social Workers, psychiatric nurses in the American Nursing Association, and employee assistance clinicians in the Employee Assistance Professional Association. Similarly, if you maintain membership in any other professional organization with an ethics code, be sure to document it. If you are not a member of any such organization, it would be worthwhile to join one. More information about these organizations can be found on the internet (www.ama-assn,org, American Medical Association; www.psych.org, American Psychiatric Association; www.apa.org, American Psychological Association; www.nasw.org, National Association of Social Workers; www.nursingworld.org, American Nursing Association; and www.eap-association.com, Employee Assistance Professionals Association).

Letters of Recommendation

Many MCOs will request several letters of recommendation from professionals familiar with your work. If at all possible, it is desirable to obtain letters of reference from colleagues already in the prospective MCO's network. In many cases this will not be possible, and a letter from a person familiar with your work will be sufficient. In many cases, the person writing the letter of recommendation will need to send the letter directly to the MCO. It is very important to follow up with anyone writing a letter of recommendation for you to make sure that it was sent, and to follow up with the MCO to make sure that it was received. Your application can easily be held up for months because a letter of recommendation was not received even though you were under the impression that your colleague sent it in weeks ago. You should also be sure to read the applications carefully to determine exactly how many letters of reference are needed and who is eligible to write the letters.

SPOTLIGHT ON

Letters of Recommendation

Many MCOs will ask providers applying to join the network to provide three letters of recommendation from professionals familiar with their work. One MCO received a completed application from a provider wishing to join its network. Upon initial review of the materials, the application and all supporting documents appeared to be present. The application was completed correctly, all documents were accounted for, nothing was soon to expire, and three letters of recommendation were present. Later on, however, during a more critical review of the materials, it was discovered that while three letters of recommendation were indeed provided, they were all written by the same person. This may have been a simple misunderstanding or the provider may not have been able to get any recommendations from other colleagues. In either case, it had a seriously negative impact on the application which was ultimately denied. The lesson is simple: MCOs carefully review all application materials, therefore, whether an application says so or not, it should be assumed that each letter of recommendation must be written by a different person.

Attestations

Many applications require you to provide several attestations on topics such as any history of loss of license, liability claims, privileges, or disciplinary actions. In addition to attestations regarding your history, applications may also ask you to attest that you have not been convicted of a felony and are not currently using illegal substances. Most applications will also require you to attest that you provided a truthful and complete application.

Provider Contract

Some applications actually include the provider contract along with the application to join the network. When it is included, you are expected to carefully read the provider contact to ensure that if you are accepted you will agree to its specifications. You are expected to complete and sign the contract and return it with the application. This is done to speed up the process once you are accepted. By doing this, the MCO will not need to send you a contract and then wait for you to review, complete, and sign it as it will have already been completed. If you are not accepted into the network, the contract is simply voided by the MCO.

Common Pitfalls That Can Delay or Ruin an Application

Now that you have a basic understanding of what is expected in your application material, you will need to be aware of common pitfalls that can delay or even ruin your application. The most common of these pitfalls include expiration of documents, untimely dating of signatures, not following directions carefully, and not being truthful in the application.

Expiration of Documents

It is very important to make sure that any materials that have expiration dates or need to be renewed such as liability insurance, licenses, and registrations will not expire within 6 months of the date your application is sent to the MCO. If any materials are going to expire within the 6-month time frame, try to renew them prior to sending in the materials if possible. If this is not possible, include a note that copies of the renewed documents will be sent immediately once they are received and then take measures to ensure that this step is not forgotten, as it will delay your application.

Untimely Dating of Signatures

Many MCOs have regulations stipulating that all signatures on the application to join the network must be dated within 30 days of receipt of the application. In more than a few instances, providers begin filling out the application with all the necessary background information and signatures first. Then they work on obtaining all the necessary materials and documentation next. This step may take several weeks. Thus by the time the application is sent to the MCO, the signatures can easily be more than 30 days old. This may not get noticed until the application ends up at the credentialing committee. Once this problem is noticed, the application cannot proceed and it may then be returned to the provider to update the signatures. If this happens to you, it may take several more months before your application can be reviewed by the credentialing committee during its next meeting. Therefore it is best to sign and date all materials on the day you send in the application.

Not Following Directions Carefully

The application process is quite involved. Make sure that you read all directions carefully and that you include all requested materials. If any doubts or questions remain once the application is prepared, call the MCO's provider relations department and ask for clarification. Even small, seemingly trivial mistakes on the application can result in long delays in the application process.

Not Being Truthful on the Application

MCOs take credentialing very seriously, and the verification process is rigorous. You should assume that all information you provide will be researched and its authenticity verified, so be sure that all information is truthful.

Tips for a Successful Application

Now that you're aware of some of the common pitfalls, follow these strategies to submit a successful application.

Don't Hide It—Explain It

Having had a claim filed against you or a suspension of certain privileges in the past does not exclude you from consideration for joining a network. However, if the application asks you to list or provide an explanation of any such claims or suspensions and no explanations are given, and the MCO uncovers any such adverse events, your application will undoubtedly be rejected. Keep in mind that most of this type of information is available in the public record, and in most if not all cases the MCO will identify it during the primary verification process. Aside from the ethical issues, it really does not pay to try to hide any past history. Instead, take the opportunity to write a letter clearly explaining any previous adverse events.

Make Copies of Everything

Prior to sending in an application, be sure to photocopy the completed application and all supporting documents that are sent along with it. This simple and seemingly obvious tip is frequently overlooked. Ensuring that all materials are copied will save a great deal of time and effort if materials are lost in the mail or by the MCO.

SPOTLIGHT ON

The Importance of Copies

A social worker was contacted 2 days before the credentialing committee was set to meet in regard to his application, which had been sent in over 1 month before. The MCO apologized to the social worker, informing him that while they had a record of receiving all of his application materials, they could no longer be found. With only 2 days before the committee was set to meet, there was no way the social worker could gather all of the information again in time. Luckily, he had made a copy of his application before sending it and simply faxed a copy to the MCO. He was soon informed that he was accepted into the MCO's network.

Check Twice, Mail Once

Applications to join networks are very involved and require strict adherence to directions. Like the old saying, "measure twice, cut once," you should "check twice, mail once." It is definitely worth the time to review your application and materials carefully several times to ensure that everything is included. If any doubts or questions remain, call the MCO's provider relations department. Its staff members should be helpful in clearing up any questions as receiving applications without errors saves them time and additional work.

Fill a Need

In most cases, you should be able to get an idea of which type of provider specialties an MCO needs to add to its network simply by reading all information available on the MCO's Web site, carefully reviewing the application, and speaking with the MCO's provider relations staff. With a little effort, you can find out which populations (e.g., children and adolescents, substance-abusing members, the seriously and persistently mentally ill, etc.) an MCO needs additional providers to treat. If you have experience working with such populations, emphasize this on your application by detailing all work experience with those populations and expressing a desire to work with them in the future. Of course, if you do not have experience working with a specific population, you should not claim a specialty working with that population. That being said, you should examine your experience and figure out the MCO's needs, and then market yourself to fill that need.

SPOTLIGHT ON

Location, Location, Location

A social worker was looking to leave her position as a hospital-based therapist to enter private practice. Prior to looking for office space to rent, she first called up the provider relations departments of the three largest MCOs in her geographical area to ask for a list of their providers. After reviewing the lists, she noted certain areas where the MCOs did not have many providers. She called the MCOs to ask if their networks were open to providers in those areas and found out that two of them were. Next she began looking for office space in that area, while at the same time applying to the MCOs. Before long she was not only accepted into the networks but was receiving a fairly steady stream of referrals from the MCOs.

Be Patient

It sounds simple, but the credentialing process is slow and sometimes quite frustrating. Try to be patient and expect that it will take several months.

After avoiding the common pitfalls, utilizing the tips presented in this chapter, and waiting through the credentialing process, one of two outcomes will result: acceptance or rejection of your application. The following sections address what to expect in each of these situations.

What to Expect if Your Application Is Accepted

If your application to join the network is accepted, you will receive written notification, generally within 6 months of receipt of the application. This notification is often accompanied by a contract (if one has not already been signed during the application process), welcome materials, and a provider manual. Keep in mind that acceptance into the network does not necessarily mean that you are now able to see all members of that MCO. In fact, you may be credentialed only to treat certain lines of business for that MCO. Before proceeding to treat MCO members, make sure you are clear on exactly which members you are now contracted with the MCO to treat.

What to Do if Your Application Is Rejected

If your application to join the network is denied, the rejection will be put in writing and sent to you, typically within 6 months of receipt of your application. Upon receiving this notification, you should inquire as to the reason for the rejection. The letter may explain why. If it does not, you should place a call to provider relations to find out why. If your application was rejected due to mistakes or omissions, you should correct them and reapply. If your application was rejected because you did not meet the criteria established for membership in the network, then you should attempt to acquire the necessary training, experience, liability insurance, and so on, after which time you should submit another application. Realistically, without attaining the minimum criteria set forth by the MCO there is little chance of joining that MCO's network.

Assuming that your application was completed and the minimum requirements were met the most common reason for rejection of an application is that the network is closed. This generally means that the MCO has reached its maximum number of providers in that geographic area. If this is the reason for rejection, it is helpful to find out if the entire network is closed or simply a given geographic area. If certain geographic areas are not closed, and it is feasible, you can consider providing services in a different area where the MCO needs providers (if the MCO is agreeable) if you can establish acceptable office space, perhaps by renting office space on an hourly basis, making it possible to see patients in the area where providers are needed. You may also want to consider joining a group practice already working in the desired area.

If the entire network is closed or relocation is not feasible, it may not be possible to join the network at this time. However, networks are ever-changing entities. They are opening and closing all the time. In most cases, providers who have been turned down in an effort to join a network end their quest after one rejection. When a network is closed, you should call back the provider relations department from time to time and ask if the network has opened. It is a good idea to learn the name of the person that answers the phone. Being cordial and pleasant on the phone may help you to develop a collegial relationship with personnel in the provider relations department. With some finesse, it may be possible to get a call from the MCO whenever the network does reopen.

SPOTLIGHT ON

Persistence

A psychologist eager to join the largest MCO in her area was disappointed when she tried to apply to the network but was informed that the network was closed. Because of the great penetration rate of the MCO in her area, she knew it was imperative that she find a way to join. She used her computer's calendar to set up a reminder for her every 3 months. On receiving the reminder, she called up the MCO and asked if the network had opened. After she spoke politely with the same staff member on several attempts, the staff member offered to call her as soon as the network opened. The psychologist used the MCO's Web site to figure out the staff member's e-mail and sent her a quick thank-you e-mail. Within a few months, the psychologist got a call that the network had opened. She applied and was accepted. Remember, be polite but persistent.

Regardless of the reason for a denial of your application, the MCO should provide in writing a phone number to call in order to appeal the decision. If you believe you have been unjustly denied entrance into the network, call and appeal the decision (the appeals process is described in detail in Chapter 7).

Summary Tips

- Identify an MCO's needs and try to fill them.
- Carefully read and fully complete the application to join the network.
- Make sure all supporting documents are included.
- Date all signatures just prior to sending in the application.
- Explain, do not hide, any past adverse events.
- Your CV should emphasize any specialties, foreign language fluencies, multicultural experience, and experience working with managed care.
- Call to verify that all materials were received by the MCO.
- Be sure that no application materials will expire within 6 months of sending in the application. If they are due to expire, send in copies of the materials as soon as they are renewed and verify that they were received.
- Make copies of all submitted materials.
- If you are a psychiatrist, consider getting multiple admitting privileges and board certification in psychiatry or neurology.
- If the network is closed, periodically call the MCO to find out if it has reopened.
- Verify that all letters of recommendation have been sent and received.
- Be sure to carry at least the minimum liability coverage required by the MCO.
- When in doubt, call the provider relations department for clarification.

CHAPTER FOUR

Maintaining a Relationship With Managed Care: The Role and Function of Provider Relations

Once you have successfully joined with an MCO to become a behavioral health provider, you should start thinking about building a lasting relationship with that MCO. For many providers, getting onto an MCO panel marks the end of a long process of credentialing and brings a comforting feeling that they can just wait for referrals to come rolling in and will only have to deal with the MCO a billing issues in the future. However, for many providers, simply joining an MCO's network will not guarantee an immediate flow of referrals. Therefore, you should look at receiving credentials not as an ending but as the beginning of your relationship with an MCO, a relationship that you will need to cultivate. To build your practice, you will need to continually work on this relationship. As you will see throughout this book, the relationship you build with an MCO is the key to generating more referrals to your practice, ensuring successful audits, becoming a preferred provider, reducing denials, and speeding up the payment process. In order to develop a valuable working relationship with an MCO you will first need to understand the provider relations department and how it can help you. This chapter explains the purpose of the provider relations department and how you can utilize the department, the provider manual, and the provider newsletter to your advantage. This chapter also details the recredentialing process and the type of information provider relations departments will expect from you as a provider.

Provider Relations

For a provider on an MCO panel, the MCO's provider relations department is the connection to the MCO. Knowing how to utilize the provider relations department will help you to make the system work for you. To do this, you must first understand the role and function of the provider relations department. Essentially, it is this department's responsibility to develop and manage the MCO's network of providers. In doing so, the department handles many functions, including member services and network development, contracting, and evaluation. Additional functions may also focus on quality improvement initiatives and utilization management.

Member services typically involve assisting MCO members to access care. This can involve providing preauthorizations for behavioral health services and answering member questions about eligibility and benefits. The provider relations department will typically have a central phone number that members can use when interested in getting connected with an outpatient provider. The department is also available to handle member questions associated with claims issues. Most MCOs will have a long list of network providers available to their members. In most cases, when a member calls an MCO to get connected with an outpatient provider, a provider relations staff member consults a list of providers in that member's geographical area (usually identified by zip code) and typically provides a minimum of three provider names and contact information to the member.

Staff members who handle these calls are often asked by members whether the provider is "good" or whether he or she knows the provider. Due to the large number of providers in most MCOs, in most cases the staff member will not be familiar with the provider personally. Therefore, anything positive you can do to become known to staff members in provider relations can increase the chances that you will get more referrals. While this is not always easy, it is possible. As you work with an MCO, look for opportunities to call the provider relations department in order to develop a professional relationship with staff members. Some possibilities include the following:

- When free materials are offered, be sure to take the time to request them and to thank the staff member for sending them to you.
- When dealing with provider relations or any other part of an MCO, be polite and friendly even if they are not.
- When you speak to people on the phone, try to remember their names so that the next time you can address them by name and casually remind them that you spoke with them previously.

- If the MCO releases any new clinical practice guidelines or informs providers of any new (or existing) quality standards, don't hesitate to call provider relations for clarification about the standard. This demonstrates that you are trying to succeed on the measure, which should motivate them to refer to you.
- If you are going on vacation or are unable to receive referrals for a limited period of time, call and notify the MCO's provider relations department, even if they have never referred anyone to you.
- If the MCO refers a member to you directly, be sure to give that member a timely appointment and let the MCO know that you took steps to speed access to accommodate the member and the MCO.

SPOTLIGHT ON

Developing a Relationship With Provider Relations

A social worker found out that the MCO for which she was a network provider was conducting telephone depression screenings of all elderly members, new mothers, and members with selected chronic medical conditions. She was currently seeing one member of the MCO, whom she was treating for generalized anxiety disorder. The woman had recently given birth to a healthy boy. The social worker asked her if she received a call from the MCO asking about how she was feeling. The member replied that she had not. The provider screened for postpartum depression as the member was at high risk, having experienced depression in the past. The social worker later contacted the MCO to inform them that this woman never received a screening call and to inquire if the MCO had any additional services to offer the woman. The MCO consequently sent educational materials about postpartum depression directly to the member. The staff member who spoke with the social worker was impressed with her concern for the member and over the next few months referred new patients to the social worker. The lesson here is to look for opportunities to speak with provider relations, particularly when you can simultaneously help your patient (received educational materials) and the MCO (ensured that the member received screening and did not fall through the cracks). Believe it or not, in most cases, word of a good provider travels fast among provider relations staff members, and these are the people who have the ability to generate new referrals for you.

The provider relations department also handles network development, contracting, and evaluation. This typically involves ensuring that the MCO has an adequate provider network to meet the clinical and geographical needs of its members. It also involves handling both the credentialing and recredentialing processes and evaluation of the provider in the network to ensure that members are treated by competent providers. Provider relations is available to handle most problems or questions that providers have, yet few providers take full advantage of this resource. Typical problems or questions handled by this department include answering questions about your provider contract and responsibilities, verifying your patient's insurance benefits, and handling all questions about billing, credentialing, or any other aspect of the process of working with managed care.

Managing quality improvement initiatives is often another responsibility of the provider relations department. This typically involves administratively monitoring all network providers' performance on a quality improvement standard. For example, the quality improvement department within BHN's (2005) provider relations department has reported that it continually assesses and monitors standards such as network accessibility, member satisfaction with providers, and time between acute inpatient discharge and follow-up outpatient appointments.

Utilization management is a function of most MCOs. Utilization management ensures that members receive high-quality services in the most efficacious and typically least restrictive setting. This involves the use of authorizations of services and outpatient treatment reviews. Communicating effectively with MCOs during utilization management is discussed further in Chapter 6.

As a provider for an MCO, you should not hesitate to take advantage of the services offered to you. Maintaining involvement with the MCO through the provider relations department will keep you informed of the future needs and directions of the MCO. If you have any questions regarding any aspect of your responsibilities to the MCO or the MCO's responsibilities to you, contact the provider relations department. Fortunately, calling or e-mailing the department is not the only way to stay connected with provider relations. This can also be done through the use of the provider manual.

The Provider Manual

The provider relations department will produce a provider manual that contains essential information specific to behavioral health providers. This manual, which is typically hundreds of pages long, is the MCO's attempt to provide easy access to all of its relevant policies and important information. The manual will be provided to you upon joining an MCO. If for some reason it is not included with your welcome materials or is not available on the Web, you should call the MCO and request that it be sent to you immediately. Due to its size and generally boring nature, few providers take the time to carefully review the provider manual.

Despite its size, you should take the time to go through the manual, as it will tell you a great deal about the MCO. Included in a provider manual are the MCO's policies for authorization of services, procedures for processing claims, and information about credentialing, recredentialing, and different departments and resources within the organization. In addition to all of the policies and standards, most provider manuals will include the organization's mission and values, clinical practice guidelines, and information about how the MCO monitors quality. Becoming familiar with these will help you to set up your practice so that you will have the best possible chance of success on the MCO's quality monitors. While the MCO's perspective on quality may be very different from your own, having success on the measures will help make you known to provider relations and will go a long way toward generating referrals.

The more MCO panels you are on, the more provider manuals you will own. Given the vast amount of information included in them, it may not be feasible for you to carefully read all of them. You should, however, be sure to keep all provider manuals handy and at a minimum use them regularly as reference manuals. Be sure also to read all included clinical practice guidelines with an eye toward figuring out exactly what steps the MCO expects you to take when treating a particular condition for which they provided a clinical practice guideline. Also look carefully for any quality improvement measures that will or could be used to rate providers. Throughout your tenure as an MCO's network provider, keep in mind that answers to most questions in the following domains can be readily found in the provider manual:

- Obtaining authorization for treatment
- Credentialing and recredentialing
- Complaints, grievances, and appeals
- Utilization review
- Determining appropriate levels of care
- Claims issues
- Access standards
- How to make referrals to other MCO providers
- Discharge planning

The Provider Newsletter

In addition to producing the provider manual, another important responsibility of MCO provider relations departments is to publish and disseminate a provider newsletter.

Most major MCOs will publish a provider newsletter two to four times per year. This newsletter allows MCOs to educate providers on information they believe to be highly important. As a provider, you can expect to be sent a copy of the newsletter in the mail automatically. Many MCOs will also post past newsletters on their Web sites for providers to view. These newsletters, typically of high production quality, contain articles written by staff members of the MCO on various topics that should be of interest to providers in the MCO's network. For example, the following is a list of newsletter article headlines from provider newsletters around the country:

Pacificare Behavioral Health, Inc. (2005a)
"Keeping Members Satisfied"
"Provider Satisfaction With PBH Utilization"
"Are You Aware That PBH Has Availability Standards?"
"Quality Improvement at Pacificare"
"Preventive Health Programs Help Members Feel Good"
"Clinical Practice Guidelines in Practice"
"How PBH Makes Authorization Decisions"
"Protecting the Privacy of Consumers"
"Recognizing ADHD"

APS Healthcare (2004)
"APS Appeals Decision Time Frames"
"Information Available to Providers on the APS Web site"

Affinity Health Plan (2004)
"Reducing Suicide Risk in Your Primary Care Practice"

Cigna Behavioral Health (2002)
"Online Treatment Request Form"
"Integrating Behavioral and Medical Care"
"Timely Access to Care"
"Provider Update Information"
"Web Claims Update"

As you can see, newsletter articles can cover a wide range of topics, though most articles will relate to your clinical practice or your administrative relationship with the MCO. Despite the high quality of these newsletters, many providers do not take the time to read them, particularly providers who may be on panels of several different MCOs and thus receive several different newsletters. Failing to read the provider newsletter results in a lost opportunity to grow your practice through managed care.

Keep in mind that MCOs are not simply putting out these newsletters out of the kindness of their hearts. Newsletters are expensive to produce, so every article you see has an important reason for being there. Many of the articles appear because an outside agency such as Medicaid or the Department of Health expects the MCO to provide information on certain topics to its providers. Often the topics are associated with quality measures used by external review agencies such as NCQA. Thus, when an article contains steps you should follow as a provider, it is likely that these steps will be monitored by the MCO. A provider reading the articles with an understanding of this will be in a good position to be successful on the measures. In addition, MCOs use their newsletter to inform providers of any relevant policy changes. If you fail to read the newsletter and are unaware of the change, you may end up being denied authorization or payment in the future.

A provider who carefully reads the newsletter will better understand what is important to the MCO and can adjust his or her practice to excel in areas the MCO is looking to improve, thus increasing the likelihood of becoming a preferred provider. For example, Pacificare Behavioral Health published a newsletter article on the topic of recognizing attention-deficit/hyperactivity disorder (ADHD). Do you think that it was a coincidence that this article appeared in the newsletter shortly after NCQA discussed releasing new quality measures for the treatment of ADHD? Probably not. A newsletter article may not mention anything about new NCQA measures, but the simple fact that the MCO is publishing an article about ADHD should signal providers that this is becoming a topic of interest for the MCO and may be used in future assessments of the quality of work done by providers in the MCO's panel. Similarly, the Cigna provider newsletter published an article in 2002 about the integration of behavioral and medical care. It was probably no coincidence that this article was published shortly after NCQA released new accreditation standards in 1999 stating that all full-service MCOs must have mechanisms in place for collaboration between primary and specialty health care providers on diagnosis and treatment issues and on the use of psychotropic medications (AFSCME, 2003). Alert providers reading that article in 2002 could have figured out that careful monitoring of feedback to PCPs would become commonplace. Providers adapting their practices at that time were in a great position to do very well during audits of PCP communication forms, thus increasing their attractiveness to the MCO.

Provider newsletters often contain articles related to the administrative requirements of working with the MCO. These articles are used to inform providers about ways to reduce the time associated with claims processing. For example, more and more MCOs are beginning to offer Web-based claim submissions and Web-based verification of patient benefits. If you do not read articles on topics such as these, you will lose the opportunity to take advantage of new systems designed to make getting paid faster and easier. Provider newsletter articles also remind you of what the MCO expects of you as a provider. This can be particularly important as these expectations can be used to assess your overall quality and may even affect your recredentialing. The list of newsletter articles above demonstrates several examples of MCOs reminding providers what is expected of them (e.g., "APS Appeals Decision Time Frames", "Are You Aware That PBH Has Availability Standards?", and "Timely Access to Care").

The provider newsletter is thus a tool to better understand the MCO and what it values in providers. Therefore, when you are reading a newsletter, keep these questions in mind:

- Why is there an article on this topic right now?
- Have there been other articles on this topic recently?
- Does the article recommend that you do something clinically or administratively?
- Are quality measures mentioned?
- Can you think of any administrative measures that could be used to track whether providers are following the recommendations in the article?
- Is the article offering anything to you?
- Does anything in the newsletter give you an excuse to contact the provider relations department so as to help yourself become known to staff members?

In addition to the newsletter, an MCO may also send out a provider alert to providers. This alert is usually a letter informing you of an important change in the MCO or its policies. After you have successfully joined with an MCO, have taken the opportunity to familiarize yourself with the provider manual, and are actually reading the provider newsletters and provider alerts, the time will soon come when you are faced with the recredentialing process.

Recredentialing

In addition to managing an MCO's network of providers and producing a comprehensive provider manual, another important role of the provider relations department is to facilitate the recredentialing process. From the moment you complete the credentialing process and become a network provider, you should work at establishing and maintaining a relationship with the MCO. Over the first year or two, hopefully you will invest the time to get to know the MCO's policies and establish a working relationship with the provider relations department. Developing this relationship is important as the recredentialing process lies before you. When you are initially credentialed by an MCO, the credentialing is typically for a period of 2 to 3 years, at which point the MCO will have you go through the recredentialing process. The good news is that the recredentialing process will not be quite as time consuming for you as the credentialing process because the MCO already has a great deal of information about you on file. The bad news is that the recredentialing process is still quite involved, and simple errors can result in long delays and even loss of credentialing. To avoid this, a review of just what to expect when going through the recredentialing process is presented in this section.

Prior to going through recredentialing, it is helpful to read all of the information on this process that is available in the provider manual. Recredentialing is fairly standard across MCOs. You can expect to receive a recredentialing packet in the mail approximately 6 months before you are due for recredentialing. One mistake common among providers is to delay completing the recredentialing process. Since MCOs provide you with the materials only 6 months before your credentialing will expire, it may be a challenge for you to provide a great deal of information and documents in a limited amount of time, especially when missing a deadline can result in an MCO decision not to renew your contract. Especially when working with an MCO that may be looking to decrease the size of its network, you never want to provide an MCO with an opportunity to remove you from its network.

Regardless of which MCO is in the process of potentially recredentialing you, you will be asked to reverify all of your previous credentialing information that is subject to change. Non-high-volume providers can expect to be mailed a recredentialing packet, which will require you to complete forms and send in other professional documentation. Just as with credentialing, you will go through the process of primary verification of your credentials. Typically, the recredentialing process will be completed within 180 days. You will once again need to demonstrate that you are licensed at the highest level in the state where you practice, that your license is not restricted, and that you are carrying at least the minimum amount of professional liability insurance required by the MCO. You are also likely to be asked to reattest to statements indicating that you are willing and able to comply with the MCO's regulations and that you are able to perform all work-related responsibilities, to certify that you have not been convicted of any felonies and are not engaged in illegal activities such as illicit drug use, and to verify that you have not been sanctioned by any federal or state payment program, nor had any malpractice claims filed against you. Many of the larger MCOs, such as MHN (2005), will also include a review of one or more of the following:

- Your patient satisfaction ratings
- Your problem resolution ratings
- The speed with which you return paperwork
- Length of time to schedule an initial appointment
- Complaints against you
- Documentation of any peer review decisions

APS Healthcare (2003) also lists other measures that many MCOs now review during the recredentialing process. These include performance on quality improvement activities and any quality-of-care issues that have been documented.

While the requirements of the recredentialing process can usually be handled via mail, many MCOs will require group practices and high-volume individual providers to undergo a site visit during the recredentialing process. In addition to providing the information already described, the site visit will likely entail a review of your office and MCO members' charts.

Once all of the materials and results on MCO measures have been obtained, the information is returned to the credentialing committee for review and approval. While going through this process, keep in mind that you have certain rights as a practitioner that most if not all MCOs will recognize. These include (but are not limited to):

- The right to review the information used in support of your recredentialing application
- The right to be notified by the MCO if any information obtained by the MCO during the verification process differs significantly from the information you provided
- The right to correct any erroneous information
- The right to confidentiality for the information obtained during the recredentialing process except as otherwise provided by law

If for any reason you feel that any of these rights have been violated, you should immediately bring it to the attention of the MCO's provider relations department.

While the credentialing and recredentialing processes may feel like an overly burdensome chore to most providers, MCOs have to take the process very seriously. Most MCOs need to demonstrate to outside regulatory agencies that not only do they ensure that only high-quality providers are admitted to their network, but they are following regulatory agency standards for credentialing and recredentialing. MCOs also have to be concerned about liability. The process of verifying all of the information requested of providers serves as an attempt by the MCO to deny access to potential providers that the MCO views as having a higher risk of incurring a liability claim in the future.

Communication Expected of You as a Provider

As you have seen, once you are a credentialed or recredentialed provider, your MCO will be communicating with you through its provider manual and provider newsletters. You must also be aware that in a variety of circumstances, the MCO will expect you to communicate information to the MCO beyond the paperwork that is generated as part of the routine day-to-day operations of working with managed care.

Although many providers focus only on areas of receiving payment and obtaining approvals as topics of communication with MCOs, you should be aware that there are other areas in which the MCO will expect you to provide timely communication. This communication falls into three categories: changes to information submitted during the credentialing or recredentialing process, adverse events, and terminating your contract as a network provider.

Changes to Credentialing or Recredentialing Information

Over time, some of the information about yourself or your practice that you submitted to the MCO during credentialing or recredentialing will change. Most likely, when such changes occur your first thought will not be to notify the MCO, especially if a couple of years have passed since you went through the credentialing or recredentialing process. However, the MCO considers it your responsibility to notify it whenever these changes do occur. Common changes include changes to your mailing, billing, or practice address, telephone number, name, or your employee identification number or Social Security number. Most MCOs will also expect you to notify them if you begin to employ a billing service.

As you will recall, the application you completed for credentialing or recredentialing also asked questions about any actions taken against you professionally and about your licensing and liability coverage. Therefore, most MCOs will expect to be notified of any of the following:

- Actions taken against your license or accreditation
- Legal actions or any other actions taken against you that could impact your delivery of service
- Initiation of bankruptcy
- Expiration of your professional liability insurance coverage
- Expiration of licenses or certifications such as DEA certificate, CDS certificate, or board certification
- Expiration of registration

Keep in mind that when your license, registration, or liability coverage expires, most MCOs will expect you to submit a copy of proof of renewal, often within 5 days of expiration. Thus you should always be aware of any impending expirations and take steps not only to prevent expiration but to notify your MCO that your license, registration, or liability coverage has been renewed.

Adverse Events

In addition to changes in your personal or practice information, most MCOs will expect you to report to the MCO any adverse incidents whenever they occur. Policies about what must be reported and when it must be reported will differ somewhat by MCO, so you should familiarize yourself with the policy by reviewing the provider manual. As a general rule, you should report adverse incidents within 24 hours of occurrence. Value Options (2005a) lists the following, nonexhaustive list of examples of adverse incidents:

- Unanticipated death from any cause
- Self-inflicted harm requiring urgent or emergency care
- Violent behavior
- Adverse treatment or medication reactions requiring urgent or emergency treatment
- Medication treatment errors requiring urgent or emergency treatment in response
- Sexual behavior occurring in a behavioral health treatment setting
- Injuries due to accidents in a behavioral health treatment setting requiring urgent or emergency treatment
- Major property damage from alleged intentional acts
- Alleged human rights violations of any kind
- Any incident involving actual or potential serious harm or threat of serious litigation

In addition to these examples, MHN (2005) requires providers to report any fatal or nearly fatal electroconvulsive therapy complications. To protect yourself, be sure you understand exactly what your MCO expects of you in terms of reporting incidents to them. Keep in mind that failing to report changes in your personal or practice information or adverse events in a timely manner can adversely affect participation in the network and may even result in claims payments being denied.

Terminating Your Contract as a Network Provider

One final situation in which you would be expected to initiate communication with an MCO is if you decide to leave your MCO's network or to no longer accept new referrals from the MCO. While you are of course able to discontinue your relationship with an MCO, you must keep in mind that you still have responsibilities to patients and in many cases to the MCO. One mistake many providers often make is to simply inform the MCO that they no longer wish to participate as a provider and then refer out all patients being seen through that MCO (Psychotherapy Finances, 2004). This practice, however, is insufficient.

If you are planning to leave an MCO's network, keep in mind that there are several steps to this process. Experts on legal and ethical issues related to clinical work have outlined several steps to be followed when you wish to leave an MCO's network (Psychotherapy Finances, 2004).

Step 1: Review Your Contract

When you joined the MCO as a provider, you signed a provider contract. Before communicating that you wish to discontinue your participation, it is a good idea to carefully review the contract that you signed. Embedded in the contract should be the required minimum notice you need to give the MCO prior to termination of your relationship. If for some reason this requirement cannot be found in your contract, you should be able to find it in the provider manual or by contacting the provider relations department. As a general rule, most MCOs allow cancellation of the provider contract by either party within 30 to 90 days. In most if not all cases, cancellation of the contract will require you to submit a brief letter in writing that is signed and dated, which specifies that you wish to terminate the provider contract.

Step 2: Determine if Your Contract Allows You to Continue Treatment

After deciding to terminate your relationship with an MCO, you will need to figure out how to ensure continued appropriate care for the MCO members that you are currently treating. If you are planning to continue treating some or all of these members on a self-pay basis instead of through the MCO, you should make sure that this practice is allowed by your contract. Review your contract and speak with provider relations prior to discussing treatment options with your patients. Once you are clear on all of the limitations of your contract, then you can discuss exactly what you can and cannot offer in terms of future treatment.

Step 3: Notify Your Patients
Once you have notified the MCO of your decision to leave the network and understand all of your responsibilities in terms of your provider contract, you will need to inform your patients. This should be done verbally and in writing. You can suggest that each patient contact the MCO to obtain additional referrals. It is also a good idea to make sure that your records for that patient are current in case information is requested by the provider who will be accepting the referral and continuing treatment.

Step 4: Ensure Continuation of Proper Treatment
Keep in mind that leaving an MCO's network does not lessen your responsibility and ethical duty to ensure your patients continue to receive appropriate care. You are responsible for helping members find alternative treatment. In some cases this may mean that you will need to continue providing care to the MCO's members at the existing managed care rates (or even less). While in most cases termination and referral can be accomplished in just a few sessions, you must make sure all of your patients are transitioned to appropriate care that fits their individual treatment needs.

Summary Tips

- Find opportunities to contact provider relations in order to develop a relationship with staff members.
- Be sure to request any materials that are offered for free by provider relations (e.g., educational materials, waiting room flyers, posters, etc.).
- Actually read the provider newsletter.
- When reading provider newsletter articles, try to read between the lines by asking, why is this article appearing at this time?
- Review the provider manual.
- Start the recredentialing process early.

- Be sure to send in proof that your license, registration, liability insurance, and so on, have been renewed prior to expiration.
- Report adverse events within 24 hours.
- Be sure you know your MCO's policy on reporting adverse events.
- Don't forget to notify the MCO if any of your personal or practice information submitted during credentialing has changed.

CHAPTER FIVE

Communicating with Managed Care: Getting Services Approved

In order to get services approved and build a successful practice within the managed care environment, you will need to learn how to communicate effectively with MCOs. This means learning to speak the language of managed care. Knowing exactly what MCOs need to hear from you in order to approve services is the key to getting paid for the valuable services that you provide. As many providers find out, delivering quality care is not always more important than knowing how to describe that care because it is the description that actually gets services approved. Along with learning how to communicate with managed care, it is important that you understand exactly what information MCOs expect from you as a network provider. The better understanding you have of what MCOs are looking for and the better you are at communicating in the language of managed care, the more financially rewarding and less time consuming your relationship will be. This chapter discusses strategies for communicating with MCOs in order to get your services approved. You will need these strategies for obtaining preauthorizations for outpatient services, writing outpatient treatment reviews and reports, writing treatment plans, and requesting testing. You should also be aware of requirements MCOs look for prior to approving inpatient treatment, as you may also find yourself in the position of advocating for inpatient services for your patient.

Obtaining Preauthorization

To provide outpatient treatment to a patient in the managed care environment, you will typically first need to obtain a preauthorization for care. The process of preauthorization establishes that the patient is actively covered by the MCO and that he or she has an active mental health or substance abuse benefit. Prior to or upon first meeting with a prospective patient, you will need to obtain a preauthorization from the MCO. Typically this will involve contacting the MCO's provider relations department or visiting the MCO's Web site if it offers preauthorizations via the Web. Typically, preauthorization will require the following information:

- Policyholder's name
- Policy number
- Patient's name, address, and date of birth

Once you have provided this information, the provider relations representative should be able to create an initial authorization and should be able to provide you with the following information:

- The member's benefit limitations
- Co-payment, deductible, and coinsurance information
- The requirements for authorization of additional sessions in the future

After the preauthorization is created, most MCOs will send a letter to you and to your patient confirming the initial number of visits authorized. While the number of sessions will vary by MCO, you can expect that approximately four to five sessions will be approved initially.

A common provider mistake is to fail to obtain a preauthorization only to find out later that the member no longer has coverage, has exhausted his or her mental health benefit, or simply that the MCO will not cover the treatment provided. In fact, many MCOs that require preauthorizations will deny a claim for administrative reasons, even if the member has coverage and care is appropriate, simply because a preauthorization was not obtained. Therefore, when working with an MCO, be sure you know the MCO's policy on preauthorizations for outpatient services. If you are unclear at all, you should consult the provider manual or call the provider relations department.

While obtaining preauthorization may seem like a hassle, few MCOs ever deny initial treatment for outpatient care, and the preauthorization helps to protect you from being denied payment later. Because so few preauthorizations get denied, there is currently a trend among MCOs to eliminate the preauthorization approval altogether. This has followed research demonstrating that doubling the total number of initial sessions authorized does not impact costs to the MCO (Compton, Cuffel, Burns, & Goldman, 2000). While the removal of the preauthorization process is convenient for you as a provider, you should not make the mistake of failing to verify your patient's eligibility and benefits, including any co-payments, prior to starting treatment. Remembering to check eligibility will increase in importance in instances in which the MCO has eliminated the preauthorization requirement, as failing to check eligibility on your own could result in you seeing a patient for many sessions before realizing that he or she does not have coverage.

Assuming that the MCO with whom you are working requires preauthorization for treatment, you will need to be prepared to provide specific reasons why your services are needed and exactly what you plan to accomplish during the initial assessment phase. During the preauthorization process, it is a good idea to indicate that you will be performing an assessment of your patient's psychiatric condition, conducting an assessment of risk, and determining severity of illness and the patient's capacity for change. You may also indicate that you will be developing specific strategies for improvement and working with the patient to develop specific goals for treatment. As you complete a preauthorization form on the Web or speak with a provider relations staff member, keep in mind that before an MCO approves any level of services from outpatient through inpatient, it is expected that the services are deemed medically necessary. It therefore benefits you to have an understanding of what it means (from the managed care perspective) to be "medically necessary." Most MCOs will base their criteria on established guidelines. For example, Excellus Blue Cross Blue Shield's Behavioral Health Policy (2005) offers the following criteria for medical necessity:

- Services are appropriate and consistent with the diagnosis and treatment of the medical condition.
- Services are required for the direct care and treatment or management of the condition.
- The condition would be adversely affected if the services were not provided.
- Services are provided in accordance with community standards of good medical practice.
- Services are not primarily for the convenience of the patient, patient's family, treating professional practitioner, or another practitioner.

- Services provided are the most economical level of care that can be safely provided.

While different MCOs may use slightly different criteria for medical necessity, you should use these standards as a guide to help shape your communication with an MCO. As an outpatient provider, your services are already likely to be deemed the most economical level of care. Therefore you will need to focus your efforts on communicating that the rest of the medical necessity criteria are met. Be sure to emphasize specifically why your services are needed, how they are consistent with your diagnosis, and how treatment can prevent the worsening of symptoms.

By following these guidelines, you should have no trouble obtaining preauthorization for your services. Keep in mind that since most MCOs provide an initial authorization for only a few sessions, in most cases you will need to go through the process of requesting an authorization for additional sessions, the key to which is the effective completion of an outpatient treatment review.

Authorization for Outpatient Mental Health Services

The preauthorization process typically results in authorization of a specific number of outpatient sessions. After these sessions are utilized, you will need to complete an outpatient treatment review (OTR). MCOs use these OTRs to determine whether additional outpatient treatment sessions should be approved. As you are now aware, MCOs will base this decision on whether or not the OTR effectively communicates that additional sessions are medically necessary. A common mistake made by providers is to wait until the last authorized session to begin the process of getting additional sessions approved. This can result in administrative delays and gaps in treatment for your patient. It is therefore strongly recommended that you assess your patient's needs and determine whether additional sessions will be needed prior to the last authorized session. In fact, as soon as you know for sure that more sessions will be needed, you should complete an OTR.

Submitting OTRs is critical to getting authorized for more sessions, and knowing how to communicate with an MCO through the OTR can easily be the difference between getting approved for more sessions and getting denied. Before completing an OTR, you need to know exactly what information the MCO is looking for and exactly how to provide it. Again, the key factor in getting further services approved is meeting criteria for medical necessity. You should review your MCO's provider manual to find out if the criteria used are presented. If the criteria

Severity of Need

1. The patient has or is being evaluated for a *DSM-IV* diagnosis on Axis I or Axis II (American Psychiatric Association, 1994).
2. The presenting behavioral, psychological, or biological dysfunctions are consistent with the *DSM-IV* on Axis I or Axis II.
3. Either:
   - The patient has at least mild symptomatic distress and/or impairment in functioning due to psychiatric symptoms and/or behavior in at least one of three spheres of functioning (occupational, scholastic, or social) that are direct results of an Axis I or Axis II disorder. This is evidenced by a specific clinical description of the symptoms or impairments consistent with a Global Assessment of Functioning (GAF) score of less than 71, or
   - The patient has a persistent *DSM-IV* illness for which maintenance treatment is required to maintain optimal symptom relief or functioning, or
   - There is clinical evidence that additional treatment sessions are required.
4. The patient is medically stable.

Intensity and Quality of Service

1. There is documentation of a five-axis *DSM-IV* diagnosis.
2. There is a medically necessary and appropriate treatment plan. This treatment plan is expected to be effective in either:
   - Alleviating the patient's distress or dysfunction in a timely manner, or
   - Achieving appropriate maintenance goals, or
   - Supporting termination.
3. The treatment plan addresses all relevant information (described later).

Need for Continued Treatment

1. Severity of need criteria are met, and
2. The treatment plan meets the intensity and quality of service criteria.

are not available, consider using the following criteria outlined by Magellan Behavioral Health (2006), which require you to demonstrate your patient's severity of need, the intensity and quality of service, and the need for continued treatment when requesting additional sessions (see chart on previous page).

As you complete OTRs, keep these general guidelines in mind so that you can write OTRs that will result in the approval of additional sessions. BHN (2005) also recommends that the following be included in all OTRs:

- The diagnosis is consistent with the stated symptoms.
- The proposed treatment plan adequately addresses the targeted symptoms.
- The medications are appropriate (if applicable).
- Some measurable improvement is documented.

When completing OTRs, you should heed these recommendations and make sure that you are able to satisfy the severity of need, intensity and quality of service, and need for continued treatment criteria listed above. Since the need for continued treatment criteria merely specifies success on the other two criteria, we focus on meeting the severity of need and intensity and quality of services requirements.

Severity of Need

To give authorization for further outpatient treatment, an MCO will need to know that your patient still needs care. Your OTRs should include a five-axis *DSM-IV* diagnosis with a GAF score, preferably less than 71. Keep in mind that a patient with a GAF of 71 or higher may be considered by an MCO as not having medically severe enough symptoms to need your services. When describing your patient's severity of dysfunction to establish medical necessity, your description should be consistent with your diagnosis and should be as specific and observable as possible. By clearly demonstrating the dysfunctions or limitations caused by the condition, you can make the case to the MCO that additional services are clearly needed. The following are examples of dysfunctions consistent with diagnoses:

Depression
- Patient experiences episodes of tearfulness at least three times per week.
- On average, patient sleeps less than 6 hours per night.
- Patient reports current suicidal ideation.
- Patient has missed at least 3 days of work per month in each of the last 6 months.

- Patient received his first-ever below average review at work.
- Patient failed five out of seven subjects on most recent report card.
- Patient has stopped showering and shaving daily.
- Patient was hospitalized for major depression in the past month.
- Patient has not engaged in any of her hobbies in over 4 weeks.
- Arguing with spouse has increased to approximately three times per week.
- Patient has not visited with extended family in over 6 months.
- Patient has not exercised in 2 months after regularly exercising three times per week for 1 year.
- Smoking has increased from one cigarette per day to one pack per day since onset of depression.
- Patient has gained 10 pounds since onset of depression.
- Patient has been unable to complete all homework assignments at least twice a week due to difficulty concentrating.

Anxiety
- Patient experiences nightmares at least three times per week.
- Due to anxiety, patient only leaves home when absolutely necessary.
- Patient has not traveled over a bridge in 3 years due to anxiety.
- Patient has not completed a recommended magnetic resonance imaging (MRI) scan due to anxiety.
- Patient missed five days of work last month due to fears of having a panic attack.
- Patient has avoided all areas where a crowd could potentially gather for over 6 years.
- Patient has been unable to travel for the past 2 years.
- Patient has not attended a social function in over 6 months.
- Patient checks all locks in home at least five times before being able to leave.
- Patient was late for work 10 times last month.
- Patient washes hands at least 30 times per day.
- Patient does not monitor blood glucose due to anxiety associated with needles.
- Patient is unable to speak in public.
- All areas such as restaurants, theaters, and any other place in which escape would be difficult are avoided.
- Patient has on average three panic attacks per week.
- Patient has on average three to five stomachaches per week.
- Patient left work three times in the past month due to anxiety.
- Anxiety prevents patient from raising hand to speak in class.

Substance Abuse
- Patient binge drinks at least twice per month.
- Patient broke nose during an accident while drinking 3 months ago.
- Patient missed 3 days of work last week due to drinking.
- Patient has experienced delirium tremens in the past month.
- Patient has lost two jobs in the past year due to the effects of drinking.
- Patient has been unable to pay all of monthly bills due to the cost of substance use.
- Patient continues to drink despite high blood glucose readings and worsening diabetes self-management.
- Patient smokes one pack of cigarettes per day.
- Patient drinks a six-pack of beer per day.
- Patient recently diagnosed with esophageal varices.
- Patient recently diagnosed with chronic pancreatitis.
- Patient recently involved in a car accident while using marijuana.

Serious and Persistent Mental Illness
- Patient experiences auditory hallucinations daily.
- Patient experiences visual hallucinations monthly.
- Patient hears command hallucinations instructing him/her to hurt self or others.
- A long history of medication nonadherence is present, particularly when not engaged in ongoing therapeutic treatment.
- Patient lost job last month.
- Patient is no longer showering and brushing teeth daily.
- Patient has not cleaned apartment in over 6 months.
- Thought insertion is experienced.
- Delusions of grandeur are currently being experienced.

ADHD/Impulse Disorders
- All classes were failed on most recent report card.
- Despite house rules, patient has been unable to clean room, put dishes away, or take out the trash.
- Patient is unable to complete all homework assignments more than once per week.
- Patient is unable to follow directions during gym class.
- Patient has made careless mistakes on every test this semester.
- At least once per day, the patient's parents must repeat instructions because he/she did not listen when spoken to directly.

- Patient has been unable to organize school notes.
- At least once a week, the patient loses an important item (e.g., toy, pen, homework).
- Patient speaks out of turn at least once every class.
- Patient blurts out answers before question is completed in class at least twice per week.

Intensity and Quality of Service

The key to demonstrating that your work meets the criteria for intensity and quality of service is to communicate that your goals for treatment are appropriate for your patient's condition and that, while your patient is showing improvement, additional treatment is clearly needed. Thus, when writing OTRs, be sure that all symptoms, dysfunctions, limitations, goals, and treatment frequency and intensity are consistent with your diagnosis. You will want to demonstrate measurable improvements that have been made to date while also emphasizing the continued need for treatment. Below are some examples of statements emphasizing both treatment progress and the need for continued treatment.

Depression
- Patient Health Questionnaire (PHQ) depression severity improved from severe to moderate.
- Episodes of tearfulness have been reduced to twice per week.
- Sleep has improved to 6 hours per night.
- Work/school attendance has improved to one missed day per month.
- Frequency of exercise has increased to once a week.
- The patient contacted a friend on the telephone for the first time in one month.
- The patient completed an activity scheduling chart.
- Agreement with the statement "I am a failure" reduced from 90% to 50%.
- All activities of daily living were completed every day this week.

Anxiety
- Subjective Units of Distress (SUDs) rating associated with riding in an elevator decreased from 90 to 50.
- The patient practices progressive muscle relaxation daily.
- Patient uses relaxation techniques when faced with anxiety-provoking stimuli.
- Hand washing has decreased from 30 to 20 times per day.
- The patient traveled alone for the first time in one year.

- The patient gave one presentation at work, despite SUDs rating of 80.
- The patient volunteered in class for the first time in 6 months, despite feeling very anxious.
- The patient drove over the Golden Gate Bridge for the first time in one year.
- The patient remained at work all week despite fears of an impending panic attack.
- An MRI exam was completed on the third attempt.
- The patient shook the hand of a coworker despite contamination concerns.
- The patient visited the Vietnam War Memorial despite an increase in nightmares prior to the visit.
- The patient told the story of a traumatic experience for the first time ever.
- Nightmares have been reduced to less than two per week.
- The patient rode in an elevator at work three times last week.

Substance Abuse
- Sobriety has been maintained for the past 3 weeks.
- At least five triggers for substance use have been identified by the patient.
- The patient has returned to work.
- All drug-related paraphernalia have been disposed of.
- The patient attended an AA meeting every day last week.
- The patient has avoided all contact with anyone associated with previous drug use for 10 days.
- The patient has not had any drinks on days he/she must drive for over 2 months.

Serious and Persistent Mental Illness
- Auditory hallucinations have been reduced to 2 days per week.
- The patient reported medication adherence for 7 of the last 10 days.
- The patient has showered and brushed teeth in 5 of the last 7 days.
- The patient cleaned apartment for the first time in 3 months.
- The patient completed a group session without interrupting other members for the first time in five group sessions.
- No command hallucinations have been experienced in the past 3 weeks.

ADHD/Impulse Disorders
- The patient's GPA has improved to 2.5.
- Classroom disruptions have been reduced to once per week.
- Completion of all homework assignments has increased to three times per week.

- The patient is now able to clean room without having to be reminded.
- The patient has not lost any important items in the past 2 weeks.
- Speaking out of turn in class has been reduced to less than twice per week.
- The patient has organized all class notes.
- The patient has not been involved in any physical altercations in the past 2 months.

The examples provided in this section are only a few of the many possible ways you can emphasize both the presence of improvement and the need for additional treatment. Keep in mind that MCOs use OTRs to make assessments about the quality of health care provided. In addition to the criteria for severity of need, and intensity and quality of services, an MCO may also use these reviews to determine if other hallmarks of quality care are evident. In order to satisfy most MCOs, you may need to answer the following questions:

- Is the intensity and frequency of treatment consistent with the diagnosis and severity of symptoms?
- Did you consult with other providers if the patient did not improve?
- Was a substance abuse assessment conducted?
- Was a suicide risk assessment conducted?
- Were alterations made to the treatment if your patient was not improving?
- Was a medication evaluation or adjustment considered in a timely manner?

SPOTLIGHT ON

Communicating Treatment Progress

Consider the following scenario. A clinician is treating a patient with a diagnosis of adjustment disorder with depressed mood. The patient is currently beginning the 1-year process of getting a divorce, was recently diagnosed with diabetes, and has a history of alcohol dependence. Now imagine that the clinician was seeing this patient once a week for 4 weeks and communicated the following information during an OTR:

(continued)

Communicating Treatment Progress (*continued*)

- Diagnosis: Adjustment disorder with depressed mood
- Frequency of treatment: 1–2x/week
- Expected duration of treatment: 1 year
- GAF = 70
- Dysfunctions: Anxiety, depressed mood, pressured speech
- Impairments: Lack of interest, worry
- Goals: Patient will report an improvement in his mood and will report a decrease in worry.

From the brief clinical description it is easy to see that this patient needs additional sessions to help address the stressful life events he is currently experiencing. However, to the MCO, based on the information reported this patient may not appear in need of services. Expecting treatment for 1 year for an adjustment disorder may not seem necessary to an MCO. One to two visits per week for a common adjustment disorder may also seem excessive, particularly if the patient has an outpatient mental health benefit of less than 60 visits per year. The GAF may seem rather high functioning, and some of the symptoms may seem inconsistent with the diagnosis.

If you were seeing the above-described patient, you would want to be sure to communicate the following in your OTR and other communications:

- This patient is at risk for alcohol relapse, particularly as depression or life stress was a trigger for alcohol abuse in the past. A clearly expressed treatment goal should be that the patient will not drink any alcohol for at least 6 months.
- This patient's recent diagnosis of diabetes may place him at higher risk for developing major depression. You should also express ways in which his depressed mood impacts his ability to manage his diabetes, which can easily result in a worsening of his medical condition.
- Document a detailed suicide assessment.
- Document a detailed substance abuse assessment.
- Be sure to list current life stressors. If you are aware of past responses to stressful life experiences that negatively impacted the patient, such as suicidal ideation or attempts, harm to others, impulsivity, substance

(*continued*)

Communicating Treatment Progress (*continued*)

abuse, or worsening of a behavioral health condition, emphasize the potential for these to reoccur and the need for continued treatment to avoid these negative consequences. You might consider a treatment goal such as "In the next 3 months, the patient will not make any threats of violence."

- You should also demonstrate an effort to work within the constraints of your patient's outpatient mental health benefit. You may need to space sessions or incorporate community resources such as AA.

The previous example highlighted a case in which a patient who clearly needed additional treatment appeared not to meet the criteria for continued treatment from the perspective of an MCO. Consider another case in which a request for more sessions was denied because the MCO determined that the quality of service was not appropriate.

SPOTLIGHT ON

Communicating Quality of Service

A patient was seen for panic disorder with agoraphobia. Initially, five sessions were authorized. Later an additional five sessions were authorized, followed by another five sessions. After 15 total sessions over five months, the therapist's request for additional sessions was denied. The OTR revealed the following:

- Treatment goal: The patient will leave her house at least once every day. This goal was not met as the patient has refused to leave the home except to come to treatment accompanied by her husband.
- No evidence of treatment techniques shown to be effective in treating panic disorder with agoraphobia.
- No evidence of a medication evaluation or recommendation to have one.
- No evidence of collaboration with other providers.

(*continued*)

Communicating Quality of Service (*continued*)

The provider in this case may have actually utilized behavioral techniques for treating panic disorder and recommended that medication be included as a treatment modality from the initial session, only to have the suggestion rejected by the patient. The therapist may have also collaborated with other providers and may have even made progress with this patient even though she has not come close to achieving her ultimate treatment goal. Remember, if you do not communicate it to the MCO, the MCO is free to conclude that the services did not happen. In a case like this, you should include other, less difficult goals that may be accomplished much earlier, such as the patient "will demonstrate a reduction in anxiety severity as measured by the Beck Anxiety Inventory." You should document the patient's refusal to accept a medication evaluation and also document that you recommended this more than once.

The bottom line is that when you are writing OTRs, you need to walk a fine line in order to get your services approved. You must emphasize your patient's need for continued treatment, clearly expressing the observable risks associated with premature termination, while also detailing measurable improvements made by the patient that support the effectiveness of your clinical work. As you do this, be sure that all of your communication is consistent. Your diagnosis should be consistent with your patient's reported symptoms. Your treatment goals should be consistent with your diagnosis, and your patient's progress should be consistent with your treatment goals.

A dilemma occurs when a patient you are treating shows marked improvement in functioning and may no longer meet the criteria for medical necessity even though you and your patient agree that further treatment is needed. How then do you get further sessions approved when the criteria are no longer met? Some providers unadvisedly exaggerate their patient's dysfunctions or limitations in order to get approved for the additional sessions. However, rather than misleading an MCO by misrepresenting your patient's condition on an OTR, you are much better off emphasizing the likelihood and severity of relapse, current level of stressors, and any other relevant clinical indicators that suggest further treatment is needed. Where appropriate, emphasize the prospect that if additional outpatient sessions are not provided, it is likely the patient will need a more intense (and expensive) level of care in the near future. When appropriate, also try to cite examples from the patient's past treatment history that strengthen your case for the need for additional treatment. Most MCOs will approve additional sessions when a clear case is made for the need for additional sessions. The following are some examples of statements outlining the need for additional sessions for members in remission for common diagnoses.

Depression
- This was the third onset of major depression, strongly suggesting the likelihood of future relapse and the need for relapse prevention skills.
- Despite remission of depressive symptoms, the patient continues to use alcohol excessively.
- During previous depressive episode, a new onset of depression occurred within 4 months of remission.
- Despite remission, patient experienced suicidal intent during most recent episode and has a history of suicide attempts, suggesting that continued monitoring for the return of suicidal ideation is needed.
- Despite remission, patient has a history of three hospitalizations for depression in past 5 years. Continued monitoring and relapse prevention are needed to avoid future return to the hospital.
- Depression, especially when recurrent, is a chronic disease requiring long-term monitoring (Lin et al., 2000; Unutzer et al., 2002).

Anxiety
- While the patient has had no panic attacks in the past 2 months, further sessions are needed to teach relapse prevention skills.
- While patient no longer meets criteria for agoraphobia, she continues to experience panic attacks at least twice per week.
- Although checking behaviors have stopped, additional treatment is needed to reduce anxiety associated with returning to work.
- Although the PTSD Checklist score is in the low range, patient continues to sleep less than 5 hours per night, with the lack of sleep negatively impacting her job performance.
- The patient's generalized anxiety disorder is in remission, but she reports significant depressive symptoms with a PHQ-9 score in the moderate range. These depressive symptoms are impacting her interpersonal relationships.
- Although panic attacks have stopped, she still has not completed the recommended MRI test.

Substance Abuse
- The goal of 3 month abstinence from cocaine has been achieved. Future sessions are needed to continue work on relapse prevention skills.
- Although sobriety has been achieved, the severity of the patient's medical injuries during previous intoxication warrant continued monitoring and relapse prevention.
- Although substance abuse is in remission, patient is currently experiencing a new onset stressor, similar to one that triggered a relapse in the past.
- Although remission has been achieved, the patient needs continued sessions to address anxiety associated with applying for a job as she attempts to reenter the work force.
- Discontinuation of treatment was associated with relapse and an inpatient hospitalization in the past, suggesting longer treatment engagement is needed.

Serious and Persistent Mental Illness
- Previous discontinuation of therapy was associated with a discontinuation of medication and lengthy hospitalizations.
- Medication adherence continues to be an issue for the patient.
- Although psychotic symptoms have stabilized, continued work is needed to eliminate substance use.
- Although patient is stable, additional sessions are needed to help the patient identify signs of a manic episode, as his previous manic episode resulted in an emergency room visit.
- Past depressive episodes resulted in suicidal ideation, suggesting that continued monitoring and psychoeducation are needed.

ADHD/Impulse Disorders
- Although behavioral problems have been significantly reduced, the patient continues to have academic problems due to organizational difficulties.
- Although the patient's ADHD is well controlled on medication, additional sessions are needed to address family issues affecting impulsivity that may also potentially reduce medication adherence.
- Although patient has not acted out violently in over 1 year, the seriousness of violent acts prior to treatment warrants continued treatment and close monitoring.
- Although the patient has greatly improved his anger control, a new life stressor, associated with feelings of anger, suggests that continued treatment and monitoring are still needed.

When making a case for continued sessions beyond achieving remission or after accomplishing all treatment goals, remember to emphasize the potential for avoiding costlier services later, such as hospitalizations, emergency room visits, worsening of medical conditions, relapses of mental health conditions, and potential future increases in risk of harm to self or others, as these are consequences that any MCO will be looking to avoid. In this situation, you may also want to consider informing the MCO that you will be spacing the visits as your patient has shown improvement.

To be successful in obtaining authorizations for additional outpatient treatment sessions, you will need to demonstrate the severity of need and the appropriate intensity and quality of the services you provide while going through the OTR process. This information gets communicated mostly through your treatment plan. Therefore, you will need to develop strategies for writing managed care–friendly treatment plans.

Treatment Plans

While writing treatment plans may feel like an unnecessary administrative task that takes away time from your clinical work, treatment plans are very important to MCOs. You can expect a great deal of emphasis on treatment plans, not only when requesting additional sessions but also during chart audits and any other possible requests for information from an MCO. When writing treatment plans, as when communicating anything to an MCO, it is important to first understand what they will be looking for from you.

BHN (2005) makes several recommendations for effective treatment plans that can be considered standards in managed care. First of all, your treatment plans should be clearly identifiable in the medical record. If you do not have a form for doing this, you should contact your MCO and ask if they have a treatment plan template or form that you can have. Second, you must document that you have reviewed the treatment plan with your patient (or parent if the patient is a minor) upon its completion and at least once every 3 months afterward. In addition, the following items should be present:

• Measurable treatment goals
• Estimated dates by which the goals will be achieved
• Specific interventions for each goal

Measurable Goals

One of the most common MCO complaints about providers with regard to treatment planning is the lack of measurable goals (Goldman, McCullouch, & Cuffel, 2003). While this may seem unnecessary, many MCOs are under pressure from outside evaluative agencies to demonstrate that treatment goals are observable. Thus you can be sure that the MCO you work with will expect you to incorporate measurable treatment goals. To communicate effectively with managed care, you must get into the practice of describing your treatment in terms of measurable goals even if you do not tend to think in those terms while providing care. For example, you may be working with a patient with dysthymia who has low self-esteem. In treatment, one of your main objectives may be to improve this man's self-esteem. Improving self-esteem is clearly an important goal and by doing so this man is likely to experience a decrease in depressive symptoms and an improved quality of life. However, in your communication with this patient's MCO, you would not want to say that your treatment goal is that "the patient's self-esteem will improve." A goal expressed this way is not measurable and is unlikely to be looked upon favorably by an MCO, even though improving self-esteem is vital to improvement in this patient's condition. Instead, you should think about observable ways in which low self-esteem limits your patient's functioning. For example, your goal could be that the patient will "attend at least one social event per month for the next 3 months," as low self-esteem has prevented him from attending social events. Even though your clinical work is around self-esteem, to communicate effectively with an MCO you must always speak in the language of managed care—and in this case that means expressing measurable goals for treatment. The following are examples of measurable treatment goals appropriate for a variety of commonly seen conditions.

Depression
- The patient will sleep for at least 7 hours per night for 7 consecutive days.
- Within 3 months, the patient will reduce episodes of crying from five times a day to less than twice a day.
- The patient will return to work.
- The patient will attend all classes for at least 1 week.
- The patient will miss less than 3 days of work in a calendar month.
- The patient will go for at least three 20-minute walks in a 1-week time period.
- The patient will attend at least three therapy appointments and one medication follow-up appointment within 60 days.

- The patient will leave home at least once every day for at least 1 month.
- The patient will complete an activity log for 1 week.
- The patient will meet with a friend outside of work at least once this month.
- The patient will complete and submit at least one job application this month.

Anxiety
- The patient will not experience any panic attacks for a period of at least 14 consecutive days.
- The patient will initiate at least one conversation at a social event.
- The patient will drive over a bridge at least once.
- The patient will complete scheduled MRI exam.
- The patient will get a lipid profile completed.
- The patient will practice progressive muscle relaxation at least five times outside of session.
- The patient will use guided imagery before going to sleep at least twice.
- The patient will complete an exposure assignment using a stimulus with a SUDs rating of 80 of higher for a period of at least 10 minutes on at least five separate occasions.
- The patient's nightmares will decrease from three times per week to once a week or less.
- The patient will give at least one public speech or toast.
- The patient will ride the elevator at work every day for at least 1 week.
- The patient will not wash hands more than three times a day for at least 2 weeks.
- The patient will practice exposure and response prevention every day for at least 30 days.

Substance Abuse Disorders
- The patient will identify at least three triggers for binge drinking.
- The patient will identify at least four instances when his drinking posed a risk of harm to himself or others.
- The patient will attend at least three AA meetings.
- The patient will achieve at least 3 months of marijuana abstinence.
- For at least three months, the patient will have no contact with individuals identified as triggers for cocaine use.
- All drug-related paraphernalia will be removed from the home.
- The patient will attend 90 AA sessions in 90 days.
- The patient will return to work.

- Six months of heroin abstinence will be achieved.
- The patient will request information about his MCO's quit smoking program.

Serious and Persistent Mental Illness
- The patient will take medication as prescribed every day for at least 20 consecutive days.
- The patient will attend the Friendship Club at least five times before deciding whether or not he wants to continue attending.
- The patient will shower and brush teeth every day for at least 30 days.
- The patient will clean apartment.
- The patient will remove hunting knife from his apartment, giving it to his brother for safekeeping.
- The patient will attend a medication evaluation appointment within 10 days.
- The patient will identify at least three warning signs of a manic episode.
- The patient will refrain from alcohol use for at least 3 months.
- The patient will agree to inform staff if he experiences any type of hallucination.
- The patient will not interrupt others who are speaking in a group more than once per group.

ADHD/Impulse Disorders
- The patient's GPA will rise to at least 2.5.
- The patient will complete all homework assignments for at least one entire week.
- The patient will get to school on time every day for at least 1 month.
- The patient will clean room.
- The patient and his family will complete a plan for earning rewards based on behavioral improvement.
- A quiet, neat, well-lit space for doing homework at home will be identified.
- The patient will shower and dress for school without any parental assistance.
- The patient will achieve at least a "satisfactory" on all behavior ratings on next report card.
- The patient will begin homework assignment within 10 minutes of agreed-upon homework start time (3:30 P.M.) at least four days per week.

As you can see, the key to writing effective treatment goals is making sure that each goal can be easily measured and observed. You should be aware that many providers, in an attempt to create measurable treatment goals, use phrases like "the patient will report" or "will not report." While such phrases can be used to create measurable goals, be careful about your phrasing as you can easily end up with a treatment plan goal such as, "The patient will not report any suicidal ideation for at least 3 months." While unintentional, a goal such as this gives the impression that the patient should not report suicidal ideation even if he or she is experiencing it, which of course would never be a goal of treatment. To avoid any misinterpretations, it is always a good idea to review your goals before communicating them to an MCO.

Creating measurable treatment plan goals is not always easy, particularly if you are not in the habit of thinking this way about cases. When trying to develop measurable goals, consider these questions:

1. Is there a minimum number of behaviors that would be acceptable (e.g., interrupting less than once per class)?
2. Do you know the frequency of a behavior's occurrence and does it need to be increased or decreased (e.g., leaving home at least once a day)?
3. Is there a desired outcome? Can the patient produce something that demonstrates improvement (e.g., obtaining a passing grade, returning to work)?
4. Is there anything that your patient's symptoms currently prevent him or her from accomplishing (e.g., returning to work)?
5. Is there a time frame for a behavior to occur or not occur (e.g., no panic attacks for 3 months)?
6. Can any internal, subjective states (e.g., self-esteem) be translated into external behaviors (e.g., apply for a new job)?
7. Can the patient improve baseline functioning (e.g., reducing impulsive spending from once a week to once a month or less)?

One strategy that is very helpful for creating measurable treatment plan goals is the incorporation of questionnaire assessments into your clinical work. By giving a questionnaire at your initial session with a patient, you essentially create a baseline. You can then readminister the assessment prior to the completion of your treatment plan. Since the patient will be in the habit of reviewing and signing a periodic treatment plan, getting the patient to complete a brief questionnaire should not prove difficult, particularly if you communicate the value of this assessment to your patient. Utilizing questionnaire data in this manner is also helpful as it provides useful information that can help guide your clinical work and clinical decisions (MacArthur Initiative on Depression and Primary Care, 2003). For example, lack of improvement on a questionnaire may signal the need for a medication evaluation, an increase in the frequency of sessions, or an adjustment in clinical approach. Using questionnaires in this way is also in keeping with managed care's increased use of outcome measures, described further in Chapter 9.

Estimating Dates for Treatment Goal Achievement

In addition to being measurable, treatment goals must include a date by which you expect the goal to be reached. You may have a range of time frames in mind for different goals—some short term and others long term. When working with managed care, in most cases it is preferable to emphasize shorter-term goals. Since treatment plans are typically required at least every 3 months, setting your dates for 3 months after the creation of a goal is likely to be desirable to most MCOs. In contrast, many MCOs view longer-term goals less favorably. For example, if you are creating treatment goals for a high school freshman you are treating for ADHD, most MCOs prefer a goal of "patient will pass all classes on his next report card" to "patient will graduate high school and apply to college" even if you know that this patient will need treatment throughout his high school years and his one reason for coming to treatment is to graduate high school and go to college. Remember, most MCOs prefer to think in terms of short-term progress instead of more long-term goals, which are likely to be viewed as very costly. Short-term goals also allow for greater demonstration of treatment progress. Thus, to communicate effectively with MCOs about treatment, you should incorporate measurable goals, and short-term dates by which the goals will be accomplished. In addition, the medical record should include specific interventions for each goal.

Specific Interventions for Each Goal

When communicating with managed care, consistency is a key to success. Once you have created time-limited measurable goals for treatment that are consistent with your diagnosis, you should also include in the medical record specific interventions that you have provided. These interventions should flow naturally from your diagnosis and treatment plan and should be clearly documented in the treatment record. The following are some examples of specific interventions consistent with diagnoses.

Depression
• Completed activity scheduling.
• Provided psychoeducation on depression.
• The technique of thought stopping was taught and practiced.

- The technique of evaluating the evidence was taught and practiced.
- Identifying negative automatic thoughts was taught.
- The downward arrow technique was used to identify core beliefs.
- Opportunities to increase activity levels were identified.
- Journaling was taught.
- Coping self-statements were created.
- Defense mechanisms were identified.
- Education on proper antidepressant medication adherence was provided.
- A follow-up visit with the patient's prescribing physician was strongly encouraged.
- Practiced expressing desires to spouse in a manner that is likely to be listened to by spouse.
- Suicidal ideation was assessed.

Anxiety
- Progressive muscle relaxation was taught and practiced.
- Deep breathing techniques were taught.
- Guided imagery was taught.
- Imaginal exposure was conducted.
- A hierarchy of feared stimuli was created.
- SUDs ratings were obtained.
- Exposure and response prevention was conducted.
- Psychoeducation on anxiety was provided.
- Education on proper antidepressant medication adherence was provided.
- A follow-up visit with the prescribing physician was strongly encouraged.
- Worry exposure was conducted.
- Assertiveness training was conducted.
- Stress inoculation training was conducted.

Substance Abuse
- Triggers for substance use were identified.
- Psychoeducation on the dangers of substance abuse was provided.
- Brief intervention was provided.
- Safe drinking limits were presented and discussed.
- Triggers for relapse were identified.
- Cue exposure was conducted.
- Behavioral strategies for avoiding triggers to substance use were provided.
- Hypnosis was conducted.

- Role-playing was used to practice strategies for refusing drugs.
- Goal setting was taught.

Serious and Persistent Mental Illness
- Social skills training was conducted.
- Problem solving skills training was conducted.
- Psychoeducation on schizophrenia was provided.
- Education on proper medication adherence was provided.
- A mental status exam was conducted.
- Evaluated activities of daily living (ADLs).
- Role-playing was used to practice social skills.
- Assessed family members' impressions of patient's behaviors and current needs.

ADHD/Impulse Disorders
- Provided psychoeducation on ADHD.
- Triggers for impulse behavior were identified.
- Physiological cues of anger were identified.
- Relaxation training was conducted.
- A token economy was created.
- Parents were taught how to create a less distracting homework environment for child.
- Patient was instructed to count to 10 as soon as an anger-provoking situation is identified.
- Distraction techniques were taught.
- Self-statements were taught and practiced.
- Stimulus control techniques were taught.

Keep in mind that not only should your medical record document your interventions designed to help your patient achieve treatment goals, it should also detail your patient's progress toward those goals. For example, if your treatment plan goal states that your "patient will identify at least three physiological cues for anger," simply indicating on your treatment plan review 3 months later that this goal was achieved is not enough. You should also document in the medical record the three or more physiological cues your patient identified in your progress notes for the session in which they were identified.

In many ways, the secret to getting approved for additional outpatient treatment services is knowing how to provide managed care with the information it needs in the format that it requires. To accomplish this, you must remember to emphasize the need for continued treatment while also establishing that improvement has already taken place. To do this effectively, you must use clear, specific, and measurable goals and outcomes. Central to all of your communication with managed care should be consistency. Your diagnosis flows from your patient's reported symptoms. Your treatment plan, your OTR, and your medical record documentation each flow from the diagnosis and are each consistent with each other. When you communicate in this manner, you stand a much greater chance of getting your outpatient services approved. While obtaining authorizations for additional outpatient sessions is by far the most common authorization process you are likely to face, it is also important to be familiar with other types of authorizations for other types of services. For example, at some point you may require an authorization to provide psychological testing services. You may also have a patient in need of hospitalization. It is therefore helpful to know the criteria used by many MCOs for approving testing and inpatient admissions.

Authorizations for Testing

Getting authorization for psychological testing can prove quite challenging, as many MCOs do not cover testing as part of their mental health benefits. The MCOs that do cover psychological testing often will cover only it under very few circumstances. In many cases, MCOs will not give much information to providers about the criteria used to judge whether psychological testing will be covered. While this information may be difficult to get, many MCOs that do cover psychological testing will use established criteria for making authorization decisions. By understanding the review process, you will know just what many MCOs will be looking for and how to present the need for testing in a manner most likely to result in an authorization.

When you first contact an MCO for authorization for testing, a review will be conducted to determine whether the MCO will cover the testing. During this review, the MCO will likely ask for much of the following information:

- Your patient's demographics
- Your patient's diagnoses, including all psychiatric conditions and co-occurring medical conditions
- Description of symptoms and functional impairment
- Your patient's clinical history and history of treatment
- The results of all assessments already completed

- The tests you are requesting authorization for and the number of hours you are requesting
- The specific clinical questions to be answered by the testing
- A description of how treatment will change based on the results

You can expect to be required to provide the above information when requesting testing. Keep in mind that the way you present this information can easily mean the difference between getting services approved or denied. Generally speaking, testing is most likely to be deemed necessary in complex cases in which the clinical question to be answered by the testing is specific and important, and the proposed testing is known to be valid for the clinical question (Pacificare Behavioral Health, 2005c; United Behavioral Health, 2004; Value Options, 2005b). Your task then is to establish that these standards are met. Even if your reviewer does not ask you specifically for all of the information listed above, you should be sure to provide all of it to the reviewer.

Communicating That Your Case Is Particularly Complex

To demonstrate the difficulty or complexity of your case, be sure to indicate the primary psychiatric diagnosis as well as all comorbid psychiatric diagnoses. In addition, be sure to include all relevant medical diagnoses. Keep in mind the following medical conditions known to complicate the diagnosis and treatment of psychiatric disorders: chronic obstructive pulmonary disease, coronary artery disease, heart failure, diabetes, Crohn's disease, renal failure, chronic pain, osteoarthritis, sleep apnea, rheumatoid arthritis, myocardial infarction, stroke, and cancer (Akechi et al., 2006; Boersma & Linton, 2006; deGroot, Anderson, Freedland, Clouse, & Lustman, 2001; Empana et al., 2006; Haba-Rubio, 2005; Hsich & Kao, 2005; Maly, Costigan, & Olney, 2005; Odden, Whooley, & Shlipak, 2005; Persoons et al., 2005; Sheffield et al., 1998; Yohannes, Roomi, Baldwin, & Connolly, 1998).

If you list any medical condition that complicates your patient's psychiatric diagnosis or treatment, you should also demonstrate that you have acquired medical information (or at the very least made significant attempts to acquire it) from medical treatment providers in order to improve your assessment of the patient's psychiatric and overall health condition. Failure to accomplish this step may result in a denial, with the MCO finding that you have not completed an adequate assessment that could have discovered the answer to your clinical question. Any other factors in addition to comorbid psychiatric and medical diagnoses that complicate the case should also be reported. For example, Axis IV of your diagnosis should include all relevant psychosocial stressors.

Communicating That Your Clinical Question Is Specific and Important

When requesting authorization for testing, you must be sure to have a very specific question that the testing will be able to answer. United Behavioral Health (2004) offers the following reasons for testing that may result in approval:

- The patient's differential diagnosis after the intake assessment remains unclear and testing will provide the needed clarification.
- There is significant uncertainty about the appropriate course of treatment or the patient has not responded to standard treatment with no clear explanation, and the results of the testing will have a timely effect on the treatment plan.
- Interview and other sources of information provide reasons to suspect the presence of cognitive or intellectual deficits that may adversely affect the patient's functioning or interfere with his or her ability to participate in or benefit from treatment. Testing will provide information not available from other sources that can verify the presence of suspected deficits.

As you can see from the wording of United Behavioral Health's recommendations, a nonspecific reason for testing, such as "for case conceptualization," is much less appropriate and is highly likely to be denied.

In addition to communicating a specific and important clinical question, you should also establish that you have exhausted all other less expensive and less time-consuming methods of achieving the answer to your clinical question. From an MCO's perspective in most situations, in-depth clinical interviews and the use of brief assessment instruments provide sufficient information for diagnosing mental health disorders and determining the most appropriate treatment. To establish that you have completed a thorough assessment but are still unable to answer your clinical question, you should obtain your patient's psychiatric and medical history, including information about over-the-counter and natural medications. You should also establish that you have obtained a family psychiatric and medical history relevant to the request for testing, and that you have obtained your patient's previous history of psychological testing and results. Remember that it is not enough just to take your patient's history. You must also communicate that you have completed a thorough assessment, even if you are not specifically asked to do so.

The following is a nonexhaustive list of brief rating scales that can be considered for use in lieu of, or at least prior to, requesting formal testing:

- Alcohol Use Disorders Identification Test (AUDIT)
- Brief Michigan Alcohol Screening Test (BMAST)
- Marital Satisfaction Questionnaire (MSQ)
- Mood Disorders Questionnaire (MDQ)
- Beck Depression Inventory-II (BDI-II)
- Edinburgh Post Natal Depression Scale
- State-Trait Anxiety Inventory (STAI)
- Symptom Checklist-90-R (SCL-90-R)
- Eating Disorders Inventory-2
- Impact of Events Scale
- Dissociative Experiences Scale
- PTSD Checklist (PCL)
- Patient Health Questionnaire-9 (PHQ-9)
- Beck Anxiety Inventory (BAI)
- Zung Anxiety Scale
- Geriatric Depression Scale (GDS)
- Life Events Questionnaire
- Yale-Brown Obsessive Compulsive Scale
- Center for Epidemiologic Studies-Depression (CESD)
- Structured Clinical Interview for the *DSM-IV-TR* (SCID)

Once you have established that you have identified a specific clinical question and that you have exhausted all means of answering your clinical question, you will next have to establish that the question is important. While the meaning of *important* is certainly debatable, in the context of managed care, *important* can be taken to mean, "Obtaining the answer to this clinical question will improve your treatment of this patient enough to justify the cost of testing" (Groth-Marnat, 1999, 2000; Piotrowski, 1999). Keep in mind that there are studies showing that in many cases there is insufficient evidence that formal psychological testing provides enough added value to justify its cost (Garb, 2003; Wood, Garb, Lilienfeld, & Nezworski, 2002). Therefore, when requesting preauthorization for psychological testing, the onus is on you to communicate to the reviewer specific ways in which treatment will be improved once the answer to your clinical question is obtained. Again, you should be sure to communicate this even if you are not asked specifically for this information by the reviewer. For example, you may request testing for a member diagnosed with PTSD because his self-report on the PCL does not appear consistent with his presentation in session nor with collateral information. In this case you may suspect malingering as this patient is also trying to get a "service connected status" through the Veterans Administration to receive compensation for having PTSD. You request permission to give the Minnesota Multiphasic Personality Inventory–2 (MMPI-2), the results of which would help you to decide whether to start this patient in a PTSD group program or to confront the patient about the possibility of malingering. This is particularly important since putting the patient in a group for PTSD could have a negative impact on the patient and on the other group members if he is malingering.

Communicating That the Proposed Testing Is Valid

When proposing psychological testing, you should make sure that the testing addresses a specific clinical question (Groth-Marnat, 1999, 2000; Meyer et al., 2001) and that any tests you recommend have psychometric properties demonstrating reliability and validity for use with your patient and your clinical question (American Educational Research Administration, 1990; Pacificare, 2005c; United Behavioral Health, 2004). Reliable tests should demonstrate evidence of interrater reliability, internal consistency, and test-retest reliability. The test must also be properly normed for the population for which you will be using it. For example, if interpretation of a test is based on a sample of college students, you should not presume the test is valid for use with an elderly patient. The validity of a test is more difficult to establish than reliability. Therefore, when making a request for psychological testing, make sure that the test you are requesting is considered valid for the patient you are treating and for the clinical question you are answering.

Providers often make the mistake of citing personal experience as justification for the validity of a test's use (Silver, 2001). This is inconsistent with evidence-based practice and with research showing little to no association between clinical experience and the validity of inferences drawn from psychological testing (Garb, 2002; Klonsky, 2002). In fact, if the test is not valid for the clinical question, conclusions drawn from testing could make the provider's judgments less valid (Garb, 2003; Garb, Wood, & Nezworski, 2001; Wood, Lilienfeld, Garb, & Nezworski, 2000; Wood, Nezworski, Garb, & Lilienfeld, 2001). Using your experience as evidence for validity is highly likely to result in a denial of testing services.

From most MCOs' perspective, most types of clinical questions can be answered with comprehensive interviewing, brief screening, and other methods that are less costly and time consuming than psychological testing. You should also keep in mind that the use of projective or objective personality testing should not be used as a primary method of ruling out *DSM-IV* diagnoses and that neuropsychological testing for the assessment of adult ADHD is generally not indicated (Adler & Cohen, 2004; Bornstein, 2001; Hunsley & Bailey, 2001). Some providers request psychological testing to evaluate psychological constructs such as ego strength. However, this type of clinical question is not specific, and testing for such questions may be viewed by an MCO as unlikely to improve clinical outcomes and thus is unlikely to be approved.

You may also have a difficult time obtaining approvals for projective tests in general. From the perspective of MCOs, many commonly used projective tests such as the Thematic Apperception Test, drawing tests, and most sentence completion tests have not been adequately standardized, and the value of their clinical information has not been empirically established. While Exner's scoring system for the Rorschach inkblot method has allowed for investigations of reliability, validity, and the establishment of norms, disagreements exist about the reliability and validity of its scales and indices (Garb et al., 2001). Concerns have also been raised that it overpathologizes respondents, particularly ethnic minorities (Garb et al., 2001; Hunsley & Bailey, 2001; Viglione & Hilsenroth, 2001; Wood et al., 2002; Wood & Lilienfeld, 1999; Wood, Lilienfeld, Nezworski, & Garb, 2001; Wood, Nezworski, et al., 2001). In addition, current scientific evidence has not shown that Rorschach results improve treatment outcomes (Bornstein, 2001; Garfield, 2000; Hunsley & Bailey, 2001; Viglione & Hilsenroth, 2001; Weiner, 2000; Wood et al., 2002; Wood & Lilienfeld, 1999; Wood, Lilienfeld, Garb, & Nezworski, 2000; Wood, Lilienfeld et al., 2001; Wood, Nezworski, Stejskal, Garren, & West, 1999).

On the other hand, there are some scenarios in which MCO approval for psychological testing is more likely (although this will vary by MCO). In cases where the self-report of the patient cannot be trusted, such as when malingering is suspected or collaborative information is not consistent with your patient's self-report, psychological testing may be authorized. However, you must make sure that you have a specific clinical question, the answer to which will improve treatment, and the psychological tests you request are valid for this type of situation. Examples of tests or scenarios include using the MMPI-2 when malingering is suspected and using the Continuous Performance Test when your patient is suspected of feigning ADHD (Quinn, 2003; Rogers, Sewell, Martin, & Vitacco, 2003).

Another scenario in which the need for psychological testing may arise is forensic, occupational, or school performance questions. Certain tests have proven validity for answering these questions; however, most MCOs will not cover occupational or forensic testing as it may be deemed not clinically necessary to diagnose or treat a psychiatric or substance abuse disorder and is therefore not covered under the member's mental health benefits. MCOs may also have a policy that educational testing should be conducted through the local board of education rather than through the health plan. It is a good idea to check your MCO's policy on these types of testing cases prior to requesting an authorization.

In terms of the amount of time you should request for testing, to increase the likelihood of approval, you should request only enough time to administer, score, and interpret the minimum number of tests needed to answer your clinical question. As a frame of reference, *Psychotherapy Finances* (2000) has reported that on average providers are able to bill MCOs for between 1 and 2.5 hours per test administered and interpreted.

If you are administering neuropsychological testing batteries as opposed to conducting psychological testing, you should keep in mind that most MCOs will authorize more hours due to the more intense and lengthy nature of the testing. Neuropsychological testing is generally defined as testing that is narrowly focused on providing information relevant to the determination of the presence of damage or dysfunction of the brain and associated functional deficits (United Behavioral Health, 2004). To increase the likelihood of authorization, follow the rule of thumb to request enough time to administer, score, and interpret the minimum number of tests needed to answer your clinical question. As another frame of reference, *Psychotherapy Finances* (2000) has reported that on average providers are able to bill MCO's for 6.7 hours per neuropsychological battery. They reported that managed care reimbursed for these tests:

- Minnesota Multiphasic Personality Inventory–2 (MMPI-2)
- Millon Clinical Multiaxial Inventory–III (MCMI-III)
- NEO Personality Inventory (NEO-PI)
- Leiter International Performance Scale

However, this list of tests is not exhaustive. The following practical recommendations are offered to providers trying to get approvals for psychological testing:

1. Have a specific clinical question to be answered by the testing.
2. Make sure that you explain how the results of your testing will lead to an improved treatment outcome, and how that improvement justifies the cost of the testing.
3. Make sure the tests you request are valid and reliable for use with your patient and your clinical question.

4. Communicate the complexity of your case and how testing will help to reduce that complexity.
5. If indications of substance abuse are present, be sure a thorough chemical dependency assessment has been conducted.
6. If medical symptoms are present, be sure a medical evaluation has been completed and that collaboration with medical providers has been established.
7. Exhaust all less-intense methods of assessment before requesting psychological testing and demonstrate how despite this thorough assessment, your clinical question has not been answered.
8. Request only enough testing to answer the clinical question. You have a better chance of obtaining authorization if you request only the amount of time needed to complete and interpret the minimum tests needed to answer your clinical question.

Authorization for Inpatient Mental Health Services

In addition to helping your patient to get authorization for testing services, if you feel the level of care warrants it, you may at some point need to help your patient obtain authorization for inpatient services. Therefore it is helpful for you to understand the criteria used by most MCOs when authorizing inpatient admissions. While different MCOs may use somewhat different standards, most will report the criteria they use in their provider manual. For example, Magellan Behavioral Health (2006) offers the following criteria for judging whether symptoms are severe enough to warrant psychiatric hospitalization (must have 1 and 2, and either 3 or 4):

1. Patient has a diagnosed mental illness that can be expected to improve with medical treatment.
2. There is a need for an individual plan of active psychiatric treatment that includes 24-hour access to psychiatric staffing.
3. The patient demonstrates imminent, serious harm to self or others.
4. The patient's condition requires an acute psychiatric assessment or intervention that if not provided in an inpatient setting would likely lead to serious, imminent, and dangerous deterioration of the patient's medical or mental health.

While Magellan's criteria may not be used by all MCOs, they provide a good example of how an MCO determines whether inpatient mental health care is medically necessary. It is a good idea to review the provider manual of any MCO you work with to identify their criteria. Understanding these criteria will then help you to present your patient's case to an MCO when you need to advocate for services you feel are needed.

Summary Tips

- Be sure to verify your patient's eligibility prior to providing services to ensure you will be paid for your treatment, even if preauthorization is not required.
- When pursuing authorization for additional sessions, be sure to communicate severity of need, intensity and quality of services, and need for additional treatment.
- Incorporate measurable treatment goals and outcomes into your communication with MCOs.
- Consider using questionnaires as part of your treatment goals as well as to monitor treatment progress.
- A GAF of 71 or higher may suggest to an MCO that treatment is not medically necessary.
- If the criteria for medical necessity are no longer met, do not misrepresent your patient's current condition. Instead, emphasize the reasons why continued treatment is needed and the likely negative consequences if treatment is discontinued too early.
- Be consistent. Your diagnosis, patient self-report, treatment plan, treatment goals, OTR, and medical record should all be consistent with one another.
- When requesting testing, you should emphasize reasons why the case is particularly difficult. You must also have a clinical question to be answered by the testing that is specific and important. The proposed testing must be valid for the clinical question and must be normed appropriately for your patient.
- Before requesting testing, be sure that you can document that you have done a thorough and complete assessment using less costly and time-consuming assessment tools.

CHAPTER SIX

Clinical Practice Issues: Reducing Liability

As a provider working within the managed care environment, you must always be aware of inherent liability issues. Common concerns of providers working in the managed care environment include threats to the therapeutic alliance, benefit limitations, confidentiality, and getting paid appropriately for services (Mechanic, 1998; Saakvitne & Abrahamson, 1994; Sabin, 1992; Tuttman, 1997). Like providers, MCOs are also very concerned about liability issues, particularly issues associated with appropriate record keeping such as the assessment and documentation of risk. In addition, MCOs want to ensure that all provider records match the treatment for which the MCO is being billed. This chapter covers common liability issues faced by providers working with managed care, followed by a discussion about fraud and abuse. Finally, information about managed care chart audits and how you can ensure successful audit outcomes are presented.

Common Liability Issues

Information on all of the possible liability issues faced by providers today could fill several books. This chapter will focus on liability issues that are most important to both providers and MCOs, specifically benefit limitations, appropriate documentation of risk, and confidentiality.

Benefit Limitations

The definition of *benefit limitations* is exactly what you would expect. Each MCO member has a health care policy. This policy defines all of the member's benefits covered by the MCO. For example, a member's outpatient mental health benefits may be limited to a certain number of visits per year (usually 20 or 60 visits). With some policies, a member may have an unlimited outpatient mental health benefit, meaning that the MCO will pay for as many visits per year as are medically necessary. In most cases, however, members will have a finite number of outpatient visits, after which the MCO will no longer pay for any additional outpatient mental health services.

The impact of benefit limitation is subject to two different interpretations depending on whether you are viewing it from the perspective of managed care or that of the professional provider. A benefit limitation from the MCO's perspective is simply a statement of the financial coverage to which a health plan member is entitled based exclusively on the terms of the insurance contract. The benefit limitation is the primary strategy by which insurance companies are able to statistically predict costs. While benefit limits are helpful to the MCO's bottom line, from the provider's perspective a benefit limit can feel quite constricting and at times even unfair.

Most providers view patients as being entitled to as much care as clinically necessary to achieve an optimal state of psychological health. From the provider's perspective, the work is done when it is done—that is, when the patient is functioning optimally. Thus, to most providers, mandates to use limited benefits wisely, albeit judiciously, appear artificial and constraining at best and arbitrary and capricious at worst. To initiate a treatment program within a context of a benefit of 10 paid sessions, for example, can feel quite constraining to many practitioners that face administrative barriers without regard to any consideration of the nature of the problem, the duration of the problem, or the skills and resources of the patient.

Managing benefit limitations is an important part of working with managed care. When you begin working with a patient, one of the first things you should do is find out the limitations of his or her benefits. You can ask patients if they know what their policy limitations are, but you should double check this with the MCO as many patients may not fully understand the details of a potentially confusing benefits package. Checking benefit limits can usually be done very easily by contacting the MCO or, if this information is available to providers online, by logging onto the MCO's Web site. In recent years, more and more MCOs have been making this information available to providers online and this trend is likely to continue. Keep in mind that even though your patient may be unaware, his or her medical and mental health benefits may be very different. For example, your patient may have no co-pays and unlimited outpatient medical appointment benefits, but a $25 co-pay and a 20-session limit for outpatient mental health benefits.

After you have identified your patient's benefit limitations, you should have a discussion about these limitations. A good time to do this is at the conclusion of the first session as you are formulating your diagnosis and discussing the extent of treatment needed. Sharing this reality of benefit limitations with your patient at the onset of treatment goes a long way toward establishing a mutual alliance in order to accomplish realistic goals with your patient. In most cases, the standard benefit of 20 outpatient visits in a calendar year is sufficient to satisfy the immediate goals of most patients. In the event that the patient or condition from which the patient suffers does not allow for reaching the complete goal in the time allotted, then it may be necessary to adopt lesser goals around maintenance or absence of regression, or additional community resources may need to be integrated into your treatment plan.

Managing benefit limitations may require you to adapt your practice patterns to the managed care context. Traditional psychotherapy often required consecutive weekly visits for a designated 50-minute hour until the patient achieved a set of objectives, even if these objectives took years to achieve. This model of care, while admirable, required considerable time and financial commitment. Managed care, on the other hand, tends to take a somewhat different approach to treatment, with mental health insurance coverage designed to provide alleviation of illness and rapid return to health. For some providers, remaining consistent with the vision of managed care may require adjustments to their practice. For example, if you are used to seeing all of your patients weekly and you have a managed care patient with a benefit of only 20 outpatient mental health appointments whom you believe you will need to see for a minimum of 6 months, you may want to consider seeing that patient every other week (if he or she is clinically stable enough to do so) as opposed to weekly. At the very least, you will need to be cognizant of the benefit limitation as you schedule sessions. For example, you may see the patient weekly at first but then switch to meeting every other week and then eventually monthly as he or she improves. Keep in mind, however, that it must always be clinical judgment that determines how often you see a patient.

As you balance clinical need and benefit limitations, always remember that once you accept a patient into care, you, not the MCO, are liable for the treatment. For example, imagine a provider seeing a suicidal patient with financial

SPOTLIGHT ON

Managing Benefit Limitations

A 55-year-old patient presented to the office of a social worker in January with the onset of a major depressive episode. This was the third such episode in the patient's life but his first attempt at treatment. When the social worker checked his benefits he found that this patient had a limit of 20 outpatient mental health sessions per year. After an initial assessment, it became clear that although suicidal ideation was not present, the depression was severe. Given the severity and chronic nature of this patient's depression, ongoing treatment and inclusion of medication in the treatment plan were necessary. This created a major challenge for the social worker, who knew that providing the needed care within the benefit limit would be difficult, particularly when medication visits with another provider would also be necessary. Rather than simply referring this patient to a psychiatrist, the social worker as part of routine practice asked the patient about his PCP. As it turned out, the social worker had worked with that PCP before and knew her to be proficient at prescribing antidepressant medication. The social worker obtained consent to speak with the PCP, helped the patient get an appointment with his PCP, and called the PCP to give her his impressions of the patient's condition, including the diagnosis. The PCP prescribed an antidepressant. The social worker collaborated with the PCP throughout the course of treatment to help improve the overall care. By having the PCP prescribe the medication instead of a psychiatrist, the visits for medication management did not count against the outpatient mental health benefit. The social worker also connected the patient with a no-cost community agency that sponsored a depression group and also directed him to Web-based resources for depression. Early in treatment, the social worker saw the patient weekly and monitored his symptom severity closely using a depression scale called the PHQ-9. As the patient improved, the social worker reduced the frequency of sessions. By the end of the year, the patient achieved remission and still had three outpatient mental health sessions left on his mental health benefit.

difficulties, a high co-pay, and a benefit limit of 10 sessions per year. The provider sees this patient once a month because of the benefit limitation, despite the fact that the severity of the patient's depression and suicidal ideation dictate that he should be seen much more frequently. In this hypothetical scenario, should any untoward event occur, it is the provider and not the MCO who will be liable and susceptible to lawsuits.

In terms of liability, a benefit limit does not mean that you must stop seeing a patient; it only means that the MCO does not have to continue paying for the treatment. You are ultimately responsible to provide the patient with care or an alternative subsidized program if the patient requires care, regardless of the ability to pay. Thus, absence of payment from an insurance company due to benefit limitation does not excuse you from either delivering continued care or making arrangements for government-subsidized services. The good news is that benefit limitations should be a problem in very few, if any, cases if you take the time at the start of treatment to confirm your patient's benefit limitations, discuss these limits with your patient, and establish a mutually agreed-upon plan for how to deal with the possible exhaustion of benefits. Part of the plan for handling the exhaustion of benefits could be that you will see the patient on a sliding scale or that you will refer him or her to a subsidized treatment program and ensure that your patient is satisfied with the referral. Providers demonstrating the ability to manage benefits are also highly attractive to MCOs, who view this as part of the provider's responsibility. However, as you and your patient manage these benefits, never forget that in terms of liability, it must be clinical judgment and not benefit limits that determines your practice patterns.

Appropriate Documentation of Risk

Appropriate documentation has many aspects. Two of the most important aspects of record keeping when working with managed care: assessment of risk and documenting risk.

Assessment of Risk

The rise of managed care in recent years has been associated with greater numbers of patients being treated in outpatient settings (as opposed to more intense levels of care) than ever before (Maltsberger, 2001). Some have suggested that suicides are more likely when managed care reviewers compel hospital discharge through termination of insurance benefits (Schouten, 1993) or refuse payment for partial hospitalization programs (Lewin, 1990). Whether or not the rise in managed care is truly associated with an increased number of suicidal patients being seen in outpatient settings, it is clear that assessment and documentation of patient risk carries with it the highest degree of potential liability for the private practitioner, making proper documentation of suicide assessment absolutely critical. In fact, a study found that the allegation of failure to properly monitor suicidal behavior resulting in completed suicide accounted for 16% of behavioral health care claims against providers (Brytan & Davis, 1997).

To protect yourself from liability, you should routinely conduct suicide assessments throughout the course of treatment. Suicide assessment should integrate and balance presenting clinical material from your patient's current and past history, data provided by additional informants, the patient's present illness and diagnosis, and relevant demographic factors that may heighten risk (Feldman & Finguerra, 2001). When conducting assessment of suicidality, keep in mind the following correlates of suicide completion (Maltsberger, 2001):

- Diagnoses: depression, alcoholism, drug abuse, schizophrenia
- Recent suicidal behavior: attempts, preparations, plans, communications to others
- Prior suicide attempts
- Isolation
- Recent loss
- Hopelessness
- Elderly, especially white males
- Family history of, or identification with, a suicide completer
- Economic losses
- Physical illness

These are important risk factors but are by no means the only risk factors. While you should be aware of them, keep in mind that each patient is different and should be evaluated thoroughly for suicide risk. This is particularly important as studies of providers working in managed care have shown that more than half of providers underdetect the presence of suicidal ideation (Beaudin, Vigil, & Weber, 2004). When working with MCO members, keep in mind that the rate of suicide completion is very high among the elderly (Conwell & Duberstein, 2001), while the rate of suicide attempts is very high among young people aged 15–24 (Minino, Arias, Kochanek, Murphy, & Smith, 2002). While most providers are well trained in assessing suicide risk, not all providers are in the practice of regularly documenting the results of their assessments in the patient's record on an ongoing basis throughout the course of treatment. Failing to do so opens you up to liability. Remember, if you did not document it, you have no way of showing that it happened.

Just as important as routine assessment of suicidal ideation is the assessment of violent thoughts. Key risk factors for violence toward others include, but are not limited to:

- Demographic factors—being male, young, or in the lowest socioeconomic class (Swanson, Holtzer, Gangu, & Jano, 1990)
- A history of previous violence (Buchanan, 1997) or impulsive behavior (VanDeCreek, 2000)
- Substance misuse (Link, Andrews, & Cullen, 1992)
- The presence of acute psychotic symptoms (Monahan, 1995) or transient mental states such as mania or violence obsessions (VanDeCreek, 2000)
- Unemployment (VanDeCreek, 2000)
- Lower IQ (VanDeCreek, 2000)

In addition to these general risk factors, a few specific risk factors for predicting imminence violence have been identified. These include but are not limited to threats to identifiable victims, access to potential victims, specific plans for violence, and premeditation including the purchase of a weapon (Oppenheimer & Swanson, 1990; VanDeCreek, 2000). Given the potential liability inherent in working with patients at risk for violence, you should be sure to regularly assess risk of violence and document the results of your assessment in the medical record.

Documentation of Risk
In terms of documenting risk assessment, when beginning work with a patient you should be sure to take a detailed history, including but not limited to information about correlates of suicide completion. The results of this history should appear in the record. Suicide assessment should be a regular part of ongoing treatment. You should regularly ask and document the answers to questions such as:

- Do you have thoughts of suicide?
- If so, are they related to current life stressors or have you had the thoughts before?
- Do you have a plan?
- Do you have access to the components of your plan (e.g., gun, pills, etc.)?

Whenever possible, obtain information from collateral sources and document this in the record. If you are treating a patient at risk for suicide, document the reasons you came to conclusions regarding your interventions in response to the suicidal risk. If, for example, you deemed that protection of your patient was not necessary, you should list all of the reasons that you decided that hospitalizing that patient was not deemed necessary.

When working with managed care, you should use the highest degree of care in documenting all risk assessments. You should also be aware of several important factors associated with risk. Some authors (Maltsberger, 2001; Phillips, Christenfeld, & Glynn, 1998) believe that alcoholic patients treated in the managed care context may have an elevated suicide risk, especially if kept in the hospital long enough to sober up but discharged to outpatient care without sufficient follow-up. As an outpatient provider, you should be aware of this risk and be sure to conduct thorough risk assessments in these and other high-risk cases.

Providers are also vulnerable to certain traps of the managed care environment. Inadequate history taking is the first major trap (Maltsberger, 2001). With all of the extra work, such as getting insurance information and completing paperwork, there is a temptation to rush through the process of history taking. This can lead to the failure to obtain history from family members or others who know the patient well, and to a shortening of the suicide risk assessment or documentation. Inadequate history can also lead to an incorrect diagnosis. Similarly, providers may fail to request and obtain records from previous providers. This information, vital to proper risk assessment, should not be overlooked.

Another trap providers fall into is overlooking changes in suicide risk. Assessing and documenting suicide risk is not a one-time event. A patient who does not seem suicidal at the first visit may become suicidal later. Similarly, a formerly suicidal patient may quickly become suicidal once again. Since you cannot tell a suicidal person by appearance, you must be sure to regularly assess and document risk throughout treatment (Maltsberger, 2001). Finally, many providers rely on the use of suicide contracts, whereby patients promise that they will not hurt themselves. Keep in mind that this promise is no guarantee and such contracts can potentially lull you into a false sense of security (Maltsberger, 2001).

The efforts of managed care to encourage patients to be seen in the least restrictive (and expensive) environment possible (e.g., outpatient instead of inpatient) make proper assessment and documentation of risk of the highest importance to providers working with managed care. While the managed care environment may create additional traps for providers, you should keep in mind that working with managed care also has several benefits when it comes to managing suicidal patients.

Many different levels of care are typically available to MCO members. Thus your options as a provider are not limited to simply outpatient therapy or hospitalization. You should take the time to learn about the different services the MCO offers (these can usually be found in the provider manual). In managing a suicidal patient, with an MCO you will likely have many other options such as partial hospitalization, case management, intensive outpatient treatment, home-based assessments, and so on. An MCO can also help to facilitate the transfer of needed clinical information to other treatment providers including medical providers. MCOs have large networks of providers who may serve as colleagues to collaborate with on difficult cases. MCOs also have emergency services available and often have crisis lines that can be utilized to help your patient in the event that you cannot be reached.

When working with managed care and all of the services and limitations they provide, never lose sight of the fact that you are liable for the treatment provided. The Employee Retirement Income Security Act (ERISA) limits the ability of injured patients to sue managed care plans. While there may be some exceptions to this, it is safest to assume that you maintain 100% of the liability when it comes to the treatment of your patients. Whether or not an MCO refuses to pay for services, you are still required to ensure appropriate care. A provider who addresses a patient's concerns about payment by offering suitable treatment alternatives may be protected from liability (see *Padock v. Chacko,* 1988), but one who appears to base treatment decisions on insurance coverage will have a difficult time defending him- or herself in court (see *Tabor v. Doctors Memorial Hospital,* 1990).

Keep in mind that your greatest asset, should a case ever be brought against you, is your documentation. Appropriate documentation is not only a good idea, it is your duty, as highlighted in the case of *Abille v. United States* (1980). Keyes (2001) lists the following risk management suggestions based on court cases involving assessment of suicidal patients:

- With consent, request and review prior treatment records.
- Require all team members to record notes and to read the notes of others.
- Speak to other team members (or collaborate with colleagues) and document discussion.
- Document concerns of family members and significant others.
- Document risk assessment at each outpatient visit.
- Document risk-benefit analysis each time you make a significant clinical decision, such as changing the level of suicide precautions.

In addition to suicide risk, you must also be aware of risk to others. *Tarasoff v. Regents of the University of California* (1974) is probably the best-known case articulating a duty for providers to warn identifiable individuals who may be harmed by a patient's actions. The application of duty to warn varies by state, so it is a good idea to familiarize yourself with cases addressing duty to warn in your own state (Felthous, 1999). Just like suicide risk, appropriate documentation of your decision to act or not to act is vitally important in reducing liability. Felthous (1999) recommends that when making critical decisions regarding the protection of others, the following questions should be considered and answers documented:

1. Is the patient dangerous to others?
2. Is the danger due to serious mental illness?
3. Is the danger imminent?
4. Is the danger targeted at identifiable victims?

When working with potentially dangerous patients, Keyes (2001) recommends using the following duty-to-warn risk management strategies:

- Discuss the limits of confidentiality with your patient, citing specific examples (document this discussion).
- Ask patients for permission to keep family members or significant others apprised of progress (document whether permission was granted or refused).
- Probe for a reasonable amount of detail in determining risk of harm to others who may be identifiable.

In addition, VanDeCreek (2000) states that determining risk relies on your demonstration of reasonableness and conscientiousness. Reasonableness is defined as making an effort to assess the risk of danger, documenting this, and reviewing it. Conscientiousness involves taking the risk seriously and being careful with patients in crisis (e.g., returning their calls, following up on missed appointments, not referring them before they are stable, and not abandoning them). Your documentation should reflect both your reasonableness and your conscientiousness.

When assessing for harm to others, keep in mind the importance of obtaining information from family members or other collateral sources, if possible. In addition to obtaining information from your patient and other important people, an adequate assessment also involves reviewing prior records for evidence of past violence or intended victims, consulting with other professionals if needed, and passing along information about risk to other treating providers (VanDeCreek, 2000). It is also strongly recommended that you document the date and time of interactions with patients at elevated risk, consultations with other professionals, and rationales for all clinical decisions made (VanDe Creek, 2000).

Confidentiality

Appropriate documentation in the medical record is essential to protecting yourself against many different types of potential liability. However, there is a temptation for providers to put too much information in the clinical record. This strategy of documenting everything that occurs in session can potentially jeopardize confidentiality. The need to document must be balanced with a need to protect confidentiality. While the medical record is the essential document for recording all activities relating to the care of your patients, you should keep in mind that the medical record can be subject to subpoena and managed care review, and therefore should contain only appropriate information. As a provider working with managed care, you should limit the material entered into your patients' records only to that which is clearly necessary to care, and you should protect these records from being divulged to anyone without your patients' freely given and informed consent.

You should be aware that the U.S. Department of Health and Human Services in compliance with the Health Insurance Portability and Accountability Act of 1996 (HIPAA) has elaborated the distinction between the *medical record* and *psychotherapy/personal notes* (American Psychiatric Association, 2002a). The medical record is a detailed account of administrative data, counseling session start and stop times, modalities and frequencies of treatment furnished, results of clinical tests, and any summary of the following items: diagnosis, functional status, the treatment plan, symptoms, prognosis, and progress (American Psychiatric Association, 2002a). The medical record allows for communication and continuity of care among other mental health specialists involved in the patient's care, while also providing for accurate and timely claims review and payment, and appropriate utilization review and quality of care evaluation. Furthermore, appropriate documentation is essential to substantiate services as medically necessary within the context of managed care. Because the medical record has the potential to be viewed by many different people, you must be careful what you write in it. A common complaint from many MCOs is that providers put personal information into the medical record instead of keeping this information limited to the psychotherapy notes.

Psychotherapy/personal notes, as defined by HIPAA, are notes by a mental health care provider that document or analyze the contents of conversation during sessions (Columbia University Medical Center, 2005). These notes may contain observations, impressions, and reminders. Psychotherapy notes are kept completely separate from the medical record and are considered the personal property of the provider who created them. In contrast to the medical record, psychotherapy/personal notes have the highest degree of privilege under HIPAA (Columbia University Medical Center, 2005). Stricter requirements apply for the release of psychotherapy notes than for medical record information. Generally speaking, specific written authorization is required for most disclosures—a general release form is not enough.

In terms of working with MCOs, the therapeutic note is optional whereas the medical record is required. As a provider working with managed care, you should utilize both the medical record and the psychotherapy note. The MCO usually has consent from its members to access the medical record. Therefore, you must treat the medical record as having potential to be a public document reviewed by clinical reviewers, auditors, regulatory agencies, and courts. While the medical record may be easily accessed by MCOs, psychotherapy notes may not. Insurance companies and other health plans may not make enrollment or eligibility of benefits contingent on a patient providing an authorization for disclosure of psychotherapy notes, and they should never ask you to provide copies of your psychotherapy notes in order to receive payment (American Psychiatric Association, 2002b). Thus, to maintain high standards of confidentiality, you should keep both appropriate medical records and separate personal, psychotherapy notes. The example on the following page highlights the difference between information appropriate for a medical record and information appropriate for a psychotherapy note.

While medical record notes and psychotherapy notes can take different forms, from the example you can see that the medical record focuses on symptoms, interventions, results of screens, and clinical decisions, whereas the psychotherapy note contains much of the contents of the clinical discussion. Clearly, information such as details about marital difficulties or unhappiness at work should be protected from outside agencies that could potentially review the chart in the future. Remember, you should only put in the medical record information that is safe to be viewed in court or by an MCO auditor. More personal, content-based information should go in your more highly privileged psychotherapy note.

When writing in a medical chart (or anyplace else), you should always take appropriate steps to ensure confidentiality for your patient. This becomes somewhat more challenging when conducting group or family therapy. Control of confidentiality among group therapy participants is difficult to guarantee. You should be sure to inform all group members of their responsibility to keep confidential matters that are discussed in the group, and of the inherent limitations associated with this process. Discussions of these issues early in the group's formation may serve to facilitate deeper discussion of issues of trust and boundaries. When writing

Example of a Portion of a Medical Record Note
(Recorded in Mr. M's Chart)

7/10/05

Mr. M was seen for an initial consultation. He reported the following symptoms, each occurring almost every day for longer than 1 month: depressed mood, diminished interest, difficulty sleeping, difficulty concentrating, psychomotor retardation, loss of weight, and diminished energy. He denied any current or past history of suicidal ideation or suicide attempts. He denied any current or past homicidal ideation. He denied any current alcohol or other substance use or past history of abuse. He denied any trauma history. He reported that he is taking Zoloft (50 mg/day) as of 7/1/05. The medication is prescribed by his PCP, Dr. Z. He meets criteria for the following diagnosis:

Axis I: Major depressive disorder, single episode
Axis II: None
Axis III: Hypertension
Axis IV: Problems in primary support group
Axis V: 60

Psychoeducation was provided on depression. The limits of confidentiality were presented. A follow-up appointment is scheduled for 7/17/05.

Psychotherapy Note (Kept Separate From Chart)

7/10/05

Mr. M was seen for an initial session. He is depressed and is having difficulties with several members of his family. He feels that these family members "get on him about stuff all the time" and that they are creating tension in his marriage. He mentioned that he and his wife separated for 3 months 1 year ago. He denied any substance use, but it will be helpful to monitor this over the course of treatment. He denied trauma history, but he may have felt uncomfortable disclosing at this time. He appears to use denial as a defense mechanism. He is also unhappy at his job.

notes for the group, no reference to other patients in a manner that renders them identifiable should be included in any chart. Keeping separate group psychotherapy notes can help protect you and your patients from having confidences inadvertently disclosed.

In family therapy, it may be most practical to keep records in one family member's chart. You must take special care, however, when releasing information on a chart for which family sessions have been provided. It may be wise to have all the involved family members sign a statement at the beginning of therapy acknowledging that the chart will contain information about them and specifying which signatures or combination thereof will be required to authorize access to the chart or release of information from it. In the event of substantial family change, such as divorce or a child's reaching maturity, particular care must be exercised not to release information inappropriately.

Working with an MCO can lull a provider into relaxing confidentiality standards if the provider feels like the MCO has easy access to all records. Don't be fooled MCOs take confidentiality issues very seriously, as should all providers. Always remember that you are responsible for maintaining confidentiality and demonstrating evidence of having done so. In accordance with HIPAA, you should maintain written policies and procedures regarding the protection and release of patient information. At a minimum, these policies and procedures should include:

- How patient records will be stored on-site and kept confidential
- How patient records will be stored off-site and kept confidential
- How patient information can be transmitted through phone, fax, or electronically
- How, when, and to whom patient information will be released
- The limits of confidentiality

Perhaps nowhere are issues of confidentiality more common than when requests for patient information are made by either the patient or an outside agency. When this happens, you should of course be sure to obtain the patient's consent in writing, place this document in the medical record, and discuss the potential consequences before releasing any information. Keep in mind that in some cases laws concerning the release of confidential mental health and substance abuse information will likely take precedence over other competing regulations. Since state law governs mental health and substance abuse confidentiality policies, it is wise to consult your particular state for appropriate legal standards. An added benefit of working with an MCO is that most will have an extensive legal department that may be able to provide guidance or clarify legal issues when faced with complex confidentiality or legal issues regarding your care for the MCO's member.

In addition to protecting yourself against liability issues, you must also be aware of the potential dangers of fraud and abuse.

Fraud and Abuse

While the exact legal definition of fraud can vary based on state law and legal interpretation, in the general context of managed care it can be referred to as an intentional deception or misrepresentation made by a provider with the knowledge that it result in some unauthorized benefit and includes any act constituting fraud under any applicable federal or state law (Georgia Department of Community Health, 2005). Abuse, as defined by Value Options (2005a), refers to any practice, direct or intentional, that is inconsistent with sound or established fiscal, business, insurance, or medical practices and results in unnecessary cost to a behavioral health benefits program. This also consists of reimbursement for services performed that are not medically necessary or that fail to meet professionally recognized standards for health care.

Issues of fraud and abuse are taken very seriously by lawmakers and law enforcement agencies external to MCOs as well as by the MCOs themselves. Provisions in the Balanced Budget Act of 1997 and HIPAA address issues of fraud and abuse in health care. A comprehensive antifraud program has also been created utilizing joint forces from the Centers for Medicare and Medicaid Services, the Department of Health and Human Services Offices of the Inspector General, the Federal Bureau of Investigation, and the U.S. Attorney's Office. In addition, many MCOs have departments dedicated to identifying and prosecuting instances of fraud and abuse. For example, Value Options (2005a) reports that it has both legal and fiduciary obligations to ensure that the funds it receives from clients, including federal and state government funding, is properly paid for services rendered by providers. To address this obligation, Value Options created its Special Investigations Unit to monitor and review claims and billings by providers to ensure that payments have been properly requested and made.

Billing Issues

Inaccurate or inappropriate billing practices are a common reason for charges of fraud and abuse against providers working with managed care. In most cases, billing inaccuracies are not due to an attempt on the provider's part to defraud insurance companies. Often, billing problems occur when providers are not aware of the proper codes under which to bill. When working with managed care, you can expect billing requirements to include the following (American Psychiatric Association, 2002b):

- Patient's name, address, date of birth, insurance information/ID number (note that if the patient is not the subscriber of the plan, then the subscriber information is provided with relationship to the patient)
- Clinician's name, ID number (i.e., Social Security numbers, EIN [Employer Identification number], or clinician's provider number) and address
- Facility where services were performed (e.g., office, hospital, clinic)
- Date(s), type, and location of service—current and planned
- Condition's date of onset (if different than date of service)
- Procedure code—CPT (current procedural terminology) code
- Charges
- Treatment planned—CPT code, including recommended or expected frequency
- Currently on psychiatric medications? Y/N
- Patient's status (voluntary, involuntary)
- Functional status (impairment: none, mild, moderate, or severe) or Axis V (GAF) current; highest in the past year; estimated GAF at treatment completion (would address treatment goal)
- Level of distress (none, mild, moderate, or severe) or Axis IV diagnosis
- Prognosis, that is, the estimated minimum duration of the treatment for which authorization is sought

Improper Coding
You should check with the MCO you are working with to make sure that you understand how to code properly when you submit claims. A list of commonly used CPT codes follows (keep in mind that codes can change over time, so check with your MCO):

90801	Psychiatric diagnostic interview
90804	Individual therapy (20–30 minutes)
90806	Individual therapy (45–50 minutes)
90847	Family therapy
90857	Group therapy
90862	Medication management

In addition to the correct CPT code, you must make sure that you submit the correct place of service code. Outpatient providers providing care for MCOs will most commonly use the following codes (again, check with your MCO as place of service codes may change over time):

11   Outpatient—office location
12   Home
22   Outpatient hospital

SPOTLIGHT ON

Improper Coding

A marriage and family therapist saw a family with an unlimited outpatient mental health benefit for 10 sessions of family therapy and then also saw one of the family members for two individual psychotherapy sessions. During an MCO audit of this family member's chart, it was discovered that the provider had submitted 12 claims for the psychotherapy services provided. All of the dates and diagnoses on the claims were consistent with the documented information in the chart. However, the MCO realized that all 12 claims were submitted with the CPT code 90847. Thus, the two individual therapy sessions were incorrectly coded as family therapy instead of individual therapy, which should have been coded 90806. It is easy to imagine how an honest mistake like this could happen. Even though this MCO's reimbursement rate for 90847 and 90806 were exactly the same, and it was clear to everyone involved in the audit that no possible attempt to defraud the MCO was made, the MCO was at liberty to determine that false billing had taken place and that the provider must return the payment for those individual psychotherapy sessions. The lesson here is simply that it is worth your while to double-check your claims for correctness and consistency. If anything is unclear to you, get clarification before submitting the claim. A little time invested in ensuring that your claims are consistent with treatment can save you aggravation and even money later.

It is very important that you submit the correct code. A simple mistake of indicating a place of service code of 21 instead of 11 would indicate to the MCO that you conducted the visit in a hospital. If you are an outpatient network provider with a private, non-hospital-based office, this would raise a red flag for the MCO and could result in a denial of payment. Thus you must be sure to understand and utilize appropriate codes to avoid unintentional abuse of the system.

Inconsistency between billing procedures and record keeping is a major reason why insurance companies recoup payments for claims following an audit, even if the inconsistencies are due to an honest mistake. One common error that results in denials is using code 90801 for more than one session per patient. This code is used for the initial interview only and not subsequent therapy sessions. Future 50-minute therapy sessions are coded 90806. Thus, it is your responsibility to ensure that the codes, time, dates, type of services provided, and diagnoses are documented in your patient's record in a manner that is consistent with the billing you submit to the MCO.

SPOTLIGHT ON

Proper Billing, Diagnosis, Fraud, and Abuse

The Arkansas Senior Medicare/Medicaid Patrol Training Materials (2005) warns auditors to be on the lookout for fraud involving improper billing for particular diagnoses. In the past, mental health providers have submitted claims for payment for psychotherapy sessions delivered to patients who have actually been in comas, have been in the late stages of Alzheimer's disease, or had other medical or mental health diagnoses that would make it practically impossible for them to benefit from psychotherapy. This is obviously unethical, fraudulent, and easily detected by an MCO.

Inaccurate Diagnosing

Another billing issue involves inaccurate diagnosis. The diagnosis you submit to the insurance company should be consistent with the diagnosis in the medical record, and consistent with your patient's actual presentation. Providers can run into trouble by either underreporting or overreporting diagnosis. At times, a provider may be tempted to overreport a diagnosis. In fact, this practice may not be uncommon, as Keefe and Hall (1999) have reported that many practitioners believe it is necessary to report treatment needs in ways to ensure certification rather than in ways that accurately depict patients' clinical profiles. For example, a provider might see a patient who does not quite meet criteria for major depressive disorder but does meet criteria for adjustment disorder with depressed mood. The provider knows that the MCO she is working with will approve more sessions for a major depressive disorder diagnosis than for an adjustment disorder diagnosis. Knowing this, she then submits claims for the patient with a major depression diagnosis and rationalizes that the patient needs the extra sessions and that he almost meets criteria for major depression. Clearly, this type of altering of diagnosis is unethical and opens a provider up to charges of fraud and abuse. During a future audit, discrepancies between clinical presentation and submitted diagnosis may be discovered, leading to actions taken by the MCO. It is simply not worth the risk to engage in overdiagnosing your patients in an attempt to get additional sessions authorized. To protect yourself, it is a good idea not only to diagnose accurately but to document the specific symptoms reported by your patient on which you based your diagnosis.

In other situations, a provider may be hesitant to document a diagnosis of a patient meeting *DSM* criteria. For example, a provider may decide to document a diagnosis of adjustment disorder with depressed mood for a patient who meets criteria for borderline personality disorder because of patient or provider concerns about the stigma of that diagnosis. Although the motives may be altruistic, engaging in this type of underdiagnosis can expose you and your patient to serious problems. If you minimize your diagnosis, your patient can be in jeopardy of not meeting the managed care medical necessity criteria for receiving treatment. Even if approved for initial sessions, the inaccurate underdiagnosis may result in a denial of future requests for additional sessions when, from the perspective of an MCO, the primary diagnosis does not warrant additional visits. This denial could then create serious barriers to your patient receiving needed care or could result in a great deal of out-of-pocket expense to your patient.

Co-Pay Issues

In addition to consistency and accuracy in diagnosing, the collection of co-pays represents another potential avenue for fraud and abuse. It is your responsibility to know each of your patient's co-pays and to collect them at every session. If your patient has a $20 co-pay and you know that he or she cannot afford it and is highly likely to drop out of care because of the co-pay, you cannot decide to simply waive the co-pay. By waiving the co-pay, you would be guilty of fraud against the MCO. On the other hand, if you are trying to collect co-payments, deductibles, or coinsurance that are overdue, you should be aware that you will not be authorized to charge interest or late fees. Rather than risk serious liability issues, you are better off calling your MCO's provider relations or case management department, discussing your concerns, and trying to work with the MCO to come to a mutually beneficial solution. Related to co-pays is the issue of balance billing. Imagine a provider who normally charges $100 per session. He joins an MCO network and agrees to accept $70 per session from the MCO. Upon seeing his first MCO member who has unlimited sessions with no co-pay, the provider charges the MCO member $30 per session in order to collect his usual $100 fee. It should come as no surprise that this practice, known as balance billing, is unethical and considered by the MCO to be fraudulent.

SPOTLIGHT ON

Co-Pay-Related Fraud

As clearly explained in the Value Options (2005a) provider manual, if you waive a member's co-pay, coinsurance, or deductible (assuming the member's benefit has one), you actually change the fee. For example, if you file a claim listing your usual fee of $90, but you decide to waive the member's $20 co-pay, your fee is only $70, in the view of the MCO. Accordingly, you have misrepresented your fee to the health plan, constituting fraud or a false statement within HIPAA.

Other Billing Issues

In addition to inaccuracies in billing and diagnosis, co-pay issues, and balance billing, other areas of billing fraud and abuse known to occur in the managed care environment include (but are not limited to):

- Inadequate resolution of overpayments
- Submitting claims for services not provided
- Duplicate billing
- Failure to return monies paid on claims known to be false or fraudulent
- Utilization of procedures or tests not approved or medically necessary
- Providing services that are not medically necessary
- Separately billing services that should be all inclusive
- Not seeing a patient for the full specified period of time billed for
- Overcharging

SPOTLIGHT ON

"Gang" Visits

Another situation in which mental health providers have gotten themselves into trouble involves "gang" visits. In this scheme, a mental health provider visits a facility such as a nursing home with many members from the same MCO. The provider then bills the MCO for 20 or so individual therapy or medication management appointments without actually furnishing any specific service to any of the members. If you see a large number of patients in a facility, be sure that not only are you delivering the care that you are submitting a claim for, make sure that you also carefully document the care that you did provide.

To protect yourself from charges of fraud or abuse, it is critical that you comply with all financial arrangements and maintain proper records, as these records will be reviewed if the MCO decides to audit you. In order to ensure compliance, you should carefully read your MCO contract before you sign it, with special attention to the sections on billable services (including missed appointments), co-payment rules, balance billing, telephone contacts, record keeping, and quality assurance activities. If you have any questions, be sure to obtain clarification from the MCO before signing the contract.

Although billing-related issues are the most common sources of fraud and abuse, you should be aware that they are not the only sources. Below is a nonexhaustive list of non-billing-related issues known to be causes of fraud and abuse:

- Failure to maintain confidentiality of records
- Receiving payments for referrals
- Failing to provide needed services
- Providing poor-quality services
- Violations of the billing contract
- Inappropriate documentation of services

Audits

A vital quality function of managed care organizations as well as state and federal agencies is to ensure proper documentation of patient care. National certification organizations such as the NCQA, JCAHO, state offices of mental health, and the Association for Quality and Research include in their accreditation process a section on medical record keeping. It should come as no surprise then that since MCOs are held accountable for the records kept by their contracted providers, you can be assured that they are prepared to hold you accountable for pristine record keeping and treatment documentation.

If you have never treated a patient with insurance coverage or governmental benefits such as Medicare or Medicaid and have never had a record requested for judicial purposes, then you may have developed a false impression that all of your record keeping is fine or that record keeping does not really need to be a high priority. You may also believe that as a conscientious provider you would never do anything that would warrant an audit of your charts by an outside agency. Beware of these types of thoughts, as they can lead to problems for you when working with managed care.

You should always keep in mind that the MCO may initiate an audit of your records at any time, even if you have never been audited before. An MCO will conduct an audit if any type of fraud or abuse is suspected, but it will also conduct audits if it has reason to think that utilization is not appropriate to the condition. For example, recently some MCOs have started to identify providers treating members for adjustment disorder for longer than 6 months without any evidence of a medication evaluation or review. While a provider may have very appropriate reasons for needing more than 6 months of treatment and not recommending a medication evaluation or review, to the MCO, administratively it appears that utilization may not be appropriate. Therefore, in addition to appropriate record keeping, keep in mind your diagnosis, time frame of treatment, and utilization of benefits. It is a good idea, to document in the chart reasons for the need for continued sessions (e.g., trying to get patient to return to work, patient still at risk for hospitalization, etc.) or lack of medication evaluation (e.g., patient refused).

You should also keep in mind that even when there is absolutely no reason for the MCO to believe that its members have received anything but the highest quality of care from you as a provider, you may still be audited. In fact, many MCOs will include a chart audit whenever a provider is going through the recredentialing process. Even if auditing during recredentialing is not the standard practice of an MCO you are working with, keep in mind that when any individual joins a health plan, among the items on the application is a consent form allowing the MCO to review that individual's medical record for quality of care or to audit records for evidence of fraud or abuse. Thus at any time an MCO may request a copy of your record for review without even needing any additional consent form signed.

If you are working with an MCO as part of a large group practice or you are considered a high-volume provider, your chances of being audited are probably greater than if you are an independent practitioner in a solo practice. Though the definition of high volume may vary by MCO, a general rule of thumb is that many MCOs, such as MHN, define a high-volume provider as someone who has received 25 or more MCO member referrals within 1 year (MHN, 2005).

Whether you are in a group practice or are a solo practitioner, it helps to know what to expect during an MCO audit. Usually a member of the MCO's provider relations department will come to your office and review the charts of patients you have seen or are seeing for that MCO. The auditor may or may not request a blinded copy of your charts. The auditor will have a tool that will yield an overall score which will be used to judge your charts. A minimum score for passing the audit will be set by the MCO. BHN, for example, uses a cutoff score of 67% compliance with standards as passing (BHN, 2005).

If for any reason you believe that the audit is inappropriate and you do not wish to comply with the MCO's request for charts, you should not simply ignore the request. Failure to supply requested information or to cooperate with an audit can result in disciplinary action against you for breach of your provider contract. Instead of ignoring the request, you should call the MCO's provider relations department upon receiving the request and explain your clinical apprehension in providing the requested information. Keep in mind that HIPAA allows the release of records to the MCO for health care payment and operations purposes and that the provider agreement you signed likely included a statement that you agree to comply with the MCO's quality, claims, and utilization management activities, so simply arguing that an audit violates confidentiality is unlikely to be successful.

Ensuring Successful Audits

Although each MCO will have its own tool for auditing charts, most such tools will be designed to look for similar elements. Keep in mind that many MCOs will make available to you exactly what they look for when they review charts as part of an audit. The tool used for auditing can often be found in the MCO's provider manual or sometimes even on its Web site. If this information is not available in either of these locations, it is a good idea to request a copy of the MCO's chart-auditing tool when you first join the network. Do not wait until you are being audited to search for this tool as it may be too late.

Generally speaking, almost all MCOs will want to make sure that your records are consistent with record-keeping principles that have been developed by such agencies as the American Health Information Management Association, the American Hospital Association, the American Peer Review Association, Blue Cross and Blue Shield Association, and the Health Insurance Association of America:

- The medical record must be clearly legible. It must be clear, specific, and detailed as to the precise actions taken and the impact of these actions.
- It must contain a record of the rationale behind treatment decisions.
- Past and present diagnoses must be accessible to the treating provider and consulting psychiatrist.
- Appropriate mental health risk factors must be identified and documented.
- The patient's progress must be documented.
- Response to treatment and change in treatment must be documented.
- Diagnosis revisions must be documented.
- Procedure codes (CPT codes) and diagnostic codes (*DSM-IV-R*) reported on the health insurance claim form or billing statement should be supported by the documentation in the record.

Adhering to these guidelines sets a firm foundation for a successful audit. While the guidelines seem simple, in practice you may find them rather challenging. For example, it is obvious that charts should be legible, yet how often have you struggled to read clinical notes written by previous providers? It is likely that you, too, may have written notes that are difficult for others to read, particularly when you are under pressure to write notes quickly because of time constraints and a very busy caseload. Also, keep in mind that what is legible to you may not be legible to an auditor. It is definitely worth your while to practice taking the time to ensure your handwriting is legible. If legibility remains a problem for you, consider investing in an electronic medical record to solve the problem of legibility. Remember, an unreadable chart is equivalent to an undocumented record, and an unreadable chart exposes you to liability with an MCO as well as in a court of law.

The principles above also stress the importance of documenting the reasons for your clinical decisions. Again, this will provide added protection for you in an audit as well as in court. For example, imagine a chart with the following documentation: "Patient reported suicidal ideation involving cutting himself. He denied any previous suicide attempts." Now imagine that the same patient was seen, but the following was documented: "Patient reported suicidal ideation and a vague plan to cut himself. He denied any previous suicide attempts. He denied owning any large knives. He also denied access to guns or other weapons. Patient was asked for and agreed to sign consent to allow for communication with his wife to discuss suicidal ideation. His wife was contacted and informed of his suicidal ideation. His wife agreed to remove any potential instruments of harm from the home and will remain with him. The prospect of hospitalization was discussed. Patient reported he would not commit suicide. Based on patient's report criteria for hospitalization were not met. A follow-up appointment was scheduled in 3 days. The number of his MCO's 24-hour crisis line was provided." Let's imagine that this member then attempted or committed suicide and the provider was audited or brought to trial. Which documentation do you think would be better in court? Remember, the better you support your clinical decisions in the medical record, the more protected you will be from liability during an audit or a trial.

In addition to the general principles for medical record documentation, an MCO chart audit is likely to check to ensure several other important characteristics. NCQA has created standards for behavioral health medical records that go beyond the general principles listed above. If you are audited by an MCO, chances are that the NCQA standards will be incorporated into the MCO's audit tool. These criteria include the following:

- **Patient identification:** Each page of the medical record should include a unique identifier, which may include patient identification number, medical record number, and name.
- **Personal data:** Personal information such as age, gender, contact information, marital status, legal status, and guardianship information (if applicable).
- **Consent forms:** Any signed consent forms should be included as part of the medical record.
- **Medication list:** Medications should be listed on a medication sheet and updated as needed with dosage changes and date the changes were made. The medication list should include all medications prescribed, the dosage of each medication, dates of all prescriptions, and information regarding adverse reactions.
- **Allergies:** Any allergies are documented or "no known allergies" is documented.
- **Problem list:** List of all of patient's behavioral health problems identified during the initial assessment.
- **Presenting problems:** Problems or symptoms identified by the patient or collateral sources that are occurring currently.
- **Record entries:** Each entry should include the date, clinician's name, clinician's professional degree, identification number (if applicable), and clinician's signature.

- **Alcohol/substance abuse history:** Substance abuse history must be clearly documented. This should also include smoking for patients 12 years and older.
- **Risk management issues:** Risk management issues such as harm to self or others must be prominently documented and updated.
- **Medical conditions:** All relevant medical conditions should be clearly documented and updated.
- **Appropriate use of consultations:** If patient problem is outside of your scope of expertise, you must document an appropriate referral.
- **Treatment plan:** The treatment plan should be clearly documented, incorporating measurable goals and clearly defined time frames. The record should include documentation of interventions consistent with treatment goals. Diagnoses, at a minimum, should be updated in treatment plans on a quarterly basis.
- **Diagnosis:** Diagnosis should be documented and consistent with presenting problems, history, mental status exam, and all other relevant information. Changes in diagnosis should be accompanied by a clear justification.
- **Date of next appointment:** The date of the patient's next appointment should be clearly documented. If no follow-up appointment is needed, the reasons for this should be given. If patient is referred to another provider, this should be clearly indicated.
- **Psychiatric history:** The record should include an account of all previous treatment with dates of treatment, names of providers, therapeutic interventions, effectiveness of past interventions, sources of clinical information, relevant family information, and consultation and evaluation reports.
- **Mental status examination (MSE):** Document the following aspects of the MSE: affect (e.g., constricted, blunted), speech (e.g., pressured, normal), mood (e.g., dysphoric), thought content (e.g., normal, paranoid), judgment (e.g., poor, fair), insight (e.g., limited, good), attention/concentration (e.g., inattentive, distractible), memory (long- and short-term), and impulse control (e.g., aggressive, volatile).
- **Information for children and adolescents:** A complete developmental history should be documented in the medical record.

In addition to these standards, some MCOs will also check to see that documentation of communication with the member's PCP is clearly evident in the chart. MCOs may also review your charts to determine how well you are documenting performance on quality measures. For example, an MCO may check the charts of members treated for major depression to determine whether a diagnosis is evident in the chart and at least three visits occurred within 3 months of diagnosis or initiation of medication. Some providers working in private practice do not maintain a medication list in a patient's chart because they do not prescribe medication. Do not make this mistake. Even if you do not prescribe medication, MCOs will expect that this information is clearly documented in the chart as it is important for you to have when treating a patient for any behavioral health condition. Also, more and more MCO audits are looking to see whether or not a patient's personal strengths have been identified in the record as well.

MCOs want to ensure that proper documentation is occurring. One possible area that can be overlooked by providers that is important to a reviewing MCO is the way in which corrections are made in the chart. As you are writing notes in charts, especially when under time pressure, it is inevitable that some mistakes such as spelling or grammatical errors will occur. When you notice an error and want to change it in the chart, most MCOs will expect you to draw a line through the incorrect information and note that the incorrect information was an error. This should include the date the correction was made and your initials. Erasing or using correction fluid or other such products should never occur in the treatment record. If you are making corrections in an electronic medical record, you must be able to indicate the identity of the person making the correction and the date of each correction made.

The prospect of an MCO audit of your charts may seem daunting. The information presented in this section gives you an idea of what most MCOs will be looking for during an audit. Do not make the mistake of waiting until you are about to be audited to start paying attention to these issues. Be proactive. As soon as you join a managed care network, try to obtain a copy of that MCO's auditing tool. This can often be found on the MCO's internet site, in its provider manual, or by requesting it directly from the provider relations department. Once you know exactly what will be looked for, it is much easier to shape your practice to meet those guidelines. Since you know what is desired, you should periodically take a random sample of your charts and audit them yourself with as objective an eye as possible to ensure that you are ready for an audit from any outside agency. This is not only good practice for working within the managed care environment, it is good practice for reducing liability within the legal context. Remember, in the unfortunate event of having an audit or a legal action brought against you, a properly documented chart may be your greatest asset.

At the completion of an MCO chart audit, you should receive a total score. This score is then usually compared to a standard and judged as either pass or fail. In the unlikely event that you fail an MCO audit, assuming no attempt to defraud or other highly serious issues were uncovered, actions are likely to take place. Many

---

SPOTLIGHT ON

Strategies for Successful Audits

1. Request a copy of the MCO's auditing tool upon joining the network.
2. Maintain appropriate records.
3. Write legibly.
4. Document reasons for your clinical decisions.
5. Keep all signed consent forms in the medical record.
6. Keep a medication log in the medical record.
7. Sign and date all notes.
8. Document communication with the PCP.
9. Identify your patients' personal strengths in the medical record.
10. Periodically audit your own charts.

---

provider relations departments develop educational programs to review deficiencies and to provide you with tools to help you correct the identified concerns. Some MCOs will also provide you with some sort of corrective action plan detailing which elements were below standard along with suggestions on how to properly complete your treatment records, while others will require you to submit your own corrective action plan addressing all concerns, typically within 30 days. If you are ever required to create your own corrective action plan for an MCO, be sure to document your understanding of the audit findings, your willingness to carry out all of the MCO's recommendations, and a time frame in which all changes will be implemented. The MCO will also schedule another audit in the near future, typically within a few months, to monitor your progress. It is of course expected that a significant improvement will be demonstrated during this second audit.

Summary Tips

- Review your patient's benefit limits at the very start of treatment and plan accordingly. You are responsible to ensure that your patient receives care even if the MCO no longer covers care.
- Develop your own system for auditing your charts to ensure your record keeping is timely, accurate, current, and updated to reflect all your actions and reasoning behind decisions.

- Document the medical record carefully and keep additional separate psychotherapy notes.
- Any mention of suicide or homicide must be taken seriously. Assessment of risk should be an ongoing part of treatment. All assessments should be documented.
- If it was not documented, it did not happen. Document all assessments of risk and reasons for clinical decisions.
- Do not over- or underdiagnose.
- Be consistent in all documents given to the MCO (e.g., billing, medical record, etc.).
- If keeping legible notes is a problem, invest in an electronic medical record.
- Carefully read your MCO contract. Know your fiduciary responsibilities to the MCO and their responsibilities to you.
- Discuss the limits of confidentiality with your patients at the start of treatment.

CHAPTER SEVEN

Rights and Responsibilities for Providers and Patients

As a provider working in the managed care environment, it is critical that you are aware of your rights. You and your patient will often have to request authorizations from the MCO for services. From time to time you may encounter a situation in which you feel the MCO has made an inappropriate denial or other determination that adversely affects you or your patient. In these situations, you have the right as well as the responsibility to challenge that MCO's decision. To do this successfully, it is helpful to have an understanding of the impact of local, state, and federal regulatory processes that the MCO works under. It is also helpful to understand that as a result of these regulatory processes you have certain rights as an MCO provider. By understanding these rights, you will be better prepared to exercise your most important right as a provider—the right to appeal an MCO's decision that you feel is unjust or file a grievance with the MCO. The strategies for making appeals and filing grievances provided in this chapter will give you the best possible chance of resolving any issues or disputes that may arise in your work with MCOs. However, should you go through the entire dispute process without a satisfactory resolution despite implementing these strategies, additional strategies for taking your appeal or grievance to an agency external to the MCO are provided in the final section of this chapter. In addition to understanding your rights, you should be aware of your responsibilities as a provider, particularly the responsibility to help your patient understand his or her mental health benefits.

The Impact of Local, State, and Federal Regulatory Processes

You may at times feel like you are at the mercy of the MCO, forced to accept all terms and conditions imposed upon you. However, this is not the case. MCOs are carefully regulated by a variety of local, state, and federal regulatory bodies. Although specific regulations differ somewhat by geographic location, these agencies protect the interests of the public, including both consumers and providers. Regardless of where an MCO is located, it is a safe bet that local, state, and federal regulators have determined that the MCO must protect certain rights of providers contracted to provide services for its members. Many MCOs even expressly state many of these provider rights. For example, BHN (2005) in its provider manual lists the following rights of providers:

- The right to voice a complaint or appeal
- The right to expect privacy and confidentiality consistent with state and federal laws
- The right to freely communicate with your clients about the treatment options available to them
- The right to a clear explanation of the requirements for completing outpatient treatment reports
- The right to know the clinical rationale used when a request is denied
- The right to receive all benefit payments for medically necessary services to which you are entitled in a timely fashion
- The right to collect any applicable deductible, co-payment, or coinsurance
- The right to membership information upon request
- The right to ask questions, make suggestions, or express concerns
- The right to close your practice to new members with prior notification

While many of these rights are simply rights associated with ethical business practices, the one right that you should understand in greater detail and may certainly be called upon to exercise in your work with managed care is your right to an appeal.

Appeals

MCOs have a process by which providers can appeal decisions made by the MCO that are felt to be unjust. Aside from believing that winning an appeal is not possible, some providers have concerns about appealing an MCO's decision for fear that the MCO will retaliate by refusing recredentialing or refusing to refer new members. These concerns are particularly important as providers concerned about being removed from an MCO's network are less likely to challenge an MCO directly and more likely to alter their cases for MCO reviewers, thus substituting covert (and quite possibly unethical) advocacy for direct (and ethical) advocacy (Wolff & Schlesinger, 2002). While provider concerns about making an appeal may be understandable, it is very unlikely if not impossible that any reputable MCO would retaliate against a provider who has made an honest appeal of a decision. In fact, many MCOs explicitly state that no actions will be taken against providers making appeals. For example, BHN (2005) states that providers have the right to participate in a member's appeal or complaint process without the threat of contract termination for such conduct.

All MCOs should have a formal appeals process to resolve problems between providers and the MCO. Generally speaking, when an MCO gives you a decision, it will also provide you with information on how you can appeal that decision. If this is not provided, it can easily be obtained from the provider relations department. In most cases, the appeals process will have at least two levels so that if you do not agree with the determination of your first appeal, you still have a second (or further) appeal available. You must keep in mind, however, that there is usually a very small window of time available for you to file an appeal. After that time passes, your appeal may be automatically denied. For example, Value Options (2005) allows 180 calendar days after a denial to initiate a level one appeal and 90 calendar days after a denial of that appeal to file a second (level two) appeal. Therefore it is very important that you file an appeal as soon as you identify an MCO decision you believe to be unjust, as your time is limited. If you fail to meet the deadline, no matter how much evidence is in your favor, your appeal can be automatically denied. The most common types of provider appeals that you should be aware of are appeals of denial of services, credentialing decisions, and provider sanctions.

Appeals of Denial of Services

Denials of services are the most common situation in which you will need to file an appeal. Appeals of MCO denials of authorization for clinical services generally fall into one of two categories: clinical appeals and administrative appeals. Clinical appeals are generally appeals of the MCO's determination that the services were not medically necessary. Administrative appeals are responses to the MCO's decisions regarding the member's benefit provisions. Administrative denials, because they are based on benefits outlined in the member's contract, are less likely than clinical denials to be overturned. In fact, Community Behavioral HealthCare Network of Pennsylvania (CBHNP, 2004) states in its provider manual that reversal of administrative denials should be regarded as an exception and will not be routinely approved without compelling evidence.

When pursuing an appeal of a denial of services, you should be aware that most MCOs have policies stating that their members should be held harmless from financial responsibility for billed charges if services are provided during the appeal of the decision. Therefore, you should review your MCO's policies to determine a course of action. Some MCOs such as BHN (2005) will allow you to enter into a fee-for-service arrangement with the member after notifying him or her that the MCO will not cover the services. Regardless of whether you are filing a clinical or administrative appeal, the process generally has at least two levels of internal review. Each level of review should be conducted by an individual or committee that is independent of and not previously involved in the original determination. In cases of clinical appeals, the independent reviewer should have training similar to that of the providers, with experience managing the condition in question.

The first step in appealing a clinical or administrative denial is making a level one appeal. During a level one appeal, you or your patient will submit any written comments, records, documents, or any other material relevant to making the case that the denial was unjust. In a clinical appeal, the case will need to be made that the services are indeed medically necessary. Typically, a staff member or committee from the MCO that has not been involved in any aspect of the case will review the appeal and all supporting documents. Once a decision about your appeal is made, it will be submitted to you in writing. In nonurgent cases, the decision will usually take between 15 and 30 calendar days of receipt of your appeal. If you are appealing a denial when you believe that denial may seriously jeopardize the life or health of your patient, you must request an expedited appeal from the MCO. Expedited appeals, because of the serious nature of the case, are handled much quicker by MCOs. A decision regarding an expedited appeal is usually completed and issued within 3 days of the appeal. Whenever you believe an MCO's denial places your patient or anyone else at risk of death or serious harm, be sure to contact the MCO and request an expedited appeal.

Regardless of whether you file an expedited appeal or a routine appeal, you will receive a written decision informing you of the outcome of the appeal. If your appeal was denied and the original decision was upheld, your written notification should also contain the reason for the decision, information about your right to further appeal, and instructions on how to request an additional level of appeal (if this information is not present, contact provider relations). This additional level of appeal is often referred to as a level two appeal. A level two appeal is similar to a level one appeal, except that all pertinent information will be reviewed by a new staff member or committee that has not been previously involved in the case. During the level two appeal, you will have the opportunity to submit any further documents relevant to your case. Decisions on level two appeals typically take 15 to 30 calendar days from the date of submission of the appeal. Keep in mind that if you appeal an administrative denial of services, such as a denial based on exhaustion of benefits, and that denial is overturned during a level one or two appeal, the MCO will often do an additional review to make sure that the request for services meets the medical necessity criteria. Thus you could win your appeal of the administrative denial but still receive a clinical denial. Therefore, before filing an appeal, you should take the time to make sure that the criteria for medical necessity are met and that your services should be covered under your patient's benefits.

The following is a list of strategies to use throughout the process of appeals. These strategies are designed to increase your chances of making a successful appeal of a clinical or administrative denial, or simply to decrease the need for an appeal in the first place:

1. Obtain preauthorizations prior to delivering services.
2. Do your research. Before appealing, review your MCO's utilization and appeals procedures. If you have any questions, contact the provider relations department.
3. Discuss with your patient exactly what information your patient will or will not allow you to provide to the MCO during the appeals process.
4. File the appeal as soon as you become aware of any determination you feel is unjust. Remember, MCOs offer strict and short time frames for filing an appeal.
5. If your case is an emergency, be sure to request an expedited appeal.
6. The appeal should include the name and member identification number of your patient as well as the dates of requested services that are the subject of the appeal (e.g., approval of an additional five outpatient therapy sessions).
7. Only include personal information that is relevant to the appeal.
8. Make photocopies (and have your patient do the same) of every document you supply to the MCO and every document the MCO supplies to you during the entire process, especially denial letters.
9. Contact the MCO to find out the MCO's policy on coverage for your services

provided during the appeals process. If you provide therapeutic services during the appeals process, the MCO should let you know if these services will be paid by the MCO if the original denial is overturned and if it is not. You should make arrangements with your patient based on this information, ensuring that your patient will not be left without needed services.

10. If your appeal is denied, file a level two appeal right away. You have a very short window of time in which to file another appeal. Keep in mind that appeals filed after the deadline are almost always, if not always, denied.

11. If your appeal is denied, keep appealing. MCOs have multiple levels of appeals. Do not let the deadlines and additional paperwork prevent you from continuing an appeal.

SPOTLIGHT ON

Appealing Denial of Services

Recently, a psychologist was treating a man over a period of 18 months for an adjustment disorder with depressed mood. The psychologist received a notice from the MCO that future sessions with this patient would be denied due to the length of treatment already provided, the lack of demonstrated progress, and the lack of evidence of any medication evaluation (as progress with therapy alone had not been demonstrated). The psychologist discussed this with her patient. Both the psychologist and the patient agreed that continued treatment was necessary, so the psychologist filed an appeal of the MCO's decision on behalf of the patient. During the appeals process, the provider submitted documentation that the patient was also being treated by an oncologist for cancer and was already on several medications that were causing rather significant side effects. This patient was understandably unwilling to start taking an antidepressant medication on top of the medications he was already taking. In addition to coping with cancer, this patient had several other significant life stressors, all of which clearly reinforced the appropriateness of continued psychotherapy without antidepressant medication. Following the level one appeal, it was determined that the denial should be overturned and the psychologist was able to continue being reimbursed for future sessions with this patient.

Appeals of Credentialing Decisions

Another common dispute involves the appeal of an MCO's adverse credentialing decision (see Chapter 3 for information on the application process). If you complete an application to become a credentialed provider of an MCO and are denied entrance to the network, you can appeal this decision even though you are not yet a member of the network. Your denial letter should provide you with the process for filing an appeal. Unsurprisingly, you will have a very short window of time in which to file the appeal. For example, BHN (2005) gives providers 30 days from the date of the written denial letter in which to file a written request for an appeal. Therefore, as soon as you receive a denial that you feel is unjust, you must begin the appeal process. Keep in mind, however, that if the MCO denies credentials due to the network being closed in your geographical area, your appeal will be very difficult to win.

The process for appealing an adverse credentialing determination is fairly standard across the industry. Typically, all information pertaining to your case will go to a provider appeals committee within the MCO. This committee may be composed of representatives from different clinical disciplines, current network providers, and staff members from the MCO. These members should have had no participation in the MCO's original decision that is currently under review. If for some reason this is not the case, you should request that no one involved in the original determination be allowed to participate in the appeal. During the appeal, you have the opportunity to provide any additional information of your choosing, but keep in mind that the committee may also request that you provide certain information of its choosing. Listed below are strategies to employ throughout the process for successfully appealing an MCO decision to deny you entrance to its network:

1. Submit your appeal as soon as you receive a written denial.
2. Provide a clearly written explanation of the reasons you believe that the MCO's decision was in error.
3. Include all documentation that supports your case.
4. Photocopy all materials you provide to the MCO and all materials they send to you.
5. Should your appeal be denied, your written notification from the MCO should include information on how to appeal this decision. If you believe that your appeal was unjustly denied, you should immediately follow the MCO's recommendations on how to file an additional level of appeal.

SPOTLIGHT ON

Appealing a Credentialing Decision

A member in a rural area needed to obtain mental health treatment for her child who was diagnosed with autism. Unable to find a provider in her area that was a member of her MCO's panel, she presented at the office of the only psychiatrist within 20 miles of where she lived with a specialty in developmental disorders. She arranged for her child to receive the needed treatment from the psychiatrist. Her MCO reported that payment to the psychiatrist would be denied because he was not a credentialed provider for that MCO. On behalf of the patient, the psychiatrist filed an appeal and documentation was provided demonstrating that treatment was needed from a specialist and that the MCO had no such specialist in the member's area. The denial was subsequently overturned and an arrangement was made for the psychiatrist to receive payment for current and future services for the member. The MCO also reached out to the psychiatrist and offered additional incentives for him to join their network as a provider as this psychiatrist's specialty was clearly needed in that geographical area.

Appeals of MCO Sanctions

In addition to appealing denials for services or denials barring you from joining an MCO's network, you could potentially need to appeal an MCO's decision to terminate you or to impose sanctions upon you as a provider. Sanctions may be imposed due to issues related to member complaints, provider conduct, or violations of MCO policies or state or federal laws or regulations. A wide range of sanctions is used by MCOs. Value Options (2005) lists several sanctions commonly used in the industry:

- Consultation: The provider is informed of alleged actions or incidents and of sanctions to be implemented if corrective action is not taken. A copy of the consultation is kept in the provider's file and appropriate educational materials are sent to the provider.
- Written warning: A written notice of the alleged action or incident is sent. Possible sanctions to be imposed if corrective action is not taken are explained. A

copy of the written warning is placed in the provider's file and the corrective action is monitored if necessary.

- Second warning/monitoring: A second written notice is sent and placed in the provider's file and his or her performance is monitored. From the results of this monitoring, the MCO may decide to suspend new member referrals, suspend new authorizations, or redirect all current members to other providers.
- Suspension: A provider is suspended from the network pending resolution of all issues. The provider is given written notice and a copy is placed in the provider's file.
- Termination: The provider is terminated from the network. The provider is given written notification and a copy is placed in the provider's file. Members currently in care are redirected to other providers as necessary. Termination is generally reserved for serious infractions such as insolvency, loss of license, limited ability to practice, and fraud.

If you receive written notification that an MCO is imposing one of these or any other type of sanction upon you, you will have the opportunity to file an appeal. Information on how to appeal will be included in the written notification. If for some reason that information is missing, contact provider relations right away. Again, there is limited time to file an appeal. There are generally at least two levels of appeal. Once you have exhausted these appeals, if you are not satisfied with the outcome, you can usually request a fair hearing process. Typically this type of request must be made within 30 days of receiving a decision on your last appeal. This time frame may be even shorter, so you must check with your MCO to make sure that you do not miss the deadline. Usually, the MCO will send you an explanation of the hearing procedures and a list of witnesses, if any will be testifying during the hearing. The reviewers in the hearing should not have had any role in any previous decisions or appeals involving your case. If for some reason the reviewers were involved in the previous decision, you should request that they be replaced by reviewers unfamiliar with your case. Listed below are several strategies for success during the fair hearing process:

1. Request the fair hearing as soon as possible to avoid missing any deadlines.
2. Carefully read the explanation of hearing procedures.
3. Find out the MCO's policy on legal representation as the MCO may have lawyer representing them during the hearing.

4. If legal representation is allowed, strongly consider having representation during the hearing.

5. Photocopy all information submitted to the MCO or received from the MCO.

SPOTLIGHT ON

Appealing Provider Sanctions

A social worker recently went through the process of appealing a sanction against her. The MCO wanted to remove her from the network because she had lost her license to practice in the state. Her plan was to argue that she was in the process of trying to get her license renewed and she expected to be licensed again in the near future. Prior to her appeal hearing, she failed to read the information about the hearing that was sent to her and thus did not notice that the MCO would have a lawyer representing it during the appeal. The social worker did not have any legal representation during the appeal. The lesson here is to always make sure you know whether or not the MCO will have legal representation during an appeal of provider sanctions. If the MCO does have legal representation, it is best that you also consider having legal representation.

The good news is that most MCOs have to report the number and types of appeals they receive to outside regulatory agencies, so they are motivated to resolve appeals quickly and early in the appeals process. Also, the multiple levels of appeal increase the likelihood that your case will eventually get to someone or some committee who may overturn the original decision in your favor. The bad news is that there are strict rules and procedures associated with the appeals process, most notably a limited time frame in which to file an appeal.

Grievances

In addition to appealing MCO decisions, you as a provider may from time to time want to express a complaint or grievance about the MCO that is not necessarily related to an MCO's decision. MCO's have procedures for members or providers to register a complaint or grievance against the MCO, which can usually be found in the provider manual and typically involve calling a specified phone number and reporting the grievance or mailing a written grievance to a specified address. Common member grievances include issues related to quality of care, access to care, and employee service. Common provider grievances include issues related to claims processing and utilization review. If after submitting a grievance you feel that your grievance was not resolved to your satisfaction, you will generally have the opportunity to file an appeal. In most cases, grievances are settled amicably through the MCO's grievance and appeal process.

In some cases, you may find that after filing a grievance or an appeal and proceeding through the multiple levels, you are still unable to achieve a satisfactory resolution to your problem or issue. When this happens, you are not out of options. Fortunately, an avenue is available to you for filing a grievance or appeal with an external agency that has considerable power over the MCO.

Dispute Resolution by External Agencies

At times it may be necessary to go beyond the MCO to resolve a dispute. In cases where you have appealed an MCO decision and have gone through the internal appeals process yet still have not achieved a satisfactory resolution, or when you have a grievance that has not been appropriately addressed, there are external agencies you can turn to for assistance. Two very important state agencies oversee the operations of MCOs: the Department of Health and the Department of Insurance. Since the contact information for each of these agencies will differ depending on your state, you will have to look up the phone number for the agency in your particular area to pursue the filing of a grievance or appeal.

Generally speaking, the Department of Health will oversee the professional and clinical practices of the MCOs in your state. In fact, the Department of Health will typically require MCOs to report results on specific indicators of quality care. Any dispute you have with an MCO related to the delivery (or denial) of care should be addressed to your state's Department of Health. The Department of Insurance, on the other hand, typically oversees many of the business practices of the MCOs in your state and will often set business standards for MCOs. For example, the Department of Insurance may dictate the standard for the amount of time allowed for the processing of clean, submitted claims, and may also set the time frame in which providers have the opportunity to file an appeal of an MCO decision. Any dispute you have with an MCO related to its business practices should be addressed to your state's Department of Insurance.

It should come as no surprise that these departments hold great power over MCOs. You can rest assured that any grievance you file with either of these organizations will be taken very seriously by the MCO. After you have filed an external grievance, the Department of Health or the Department of Insurance will likely contact the MCO directly to inquire about the dispute. The external agency will then give the MCO a time frame to respond to the grievance and to get a resolution, which must then be reported to that agency. In most cases, you should first exhaust your internal appeals before approaching an external agency. While this may not always be possible, doing so demonstrates to the external agency that you have done all that you could to obtain a reasonable resolution within the rules set up by the MCO but have been unable to achieve a satisfactory outcome. This places greater pressure on the MCO to come up with a resolution that you will find agreeable.

If you or your patient have filed an external grievance with the Department of Health or the Department of Insurance and have still been unable to achieve an amicable resolution, you may consider recommending that your patient contact the National Mental Health Association's State Healthcare Reform Advocacy Resource Center (703-838-7524), which may be able to provide him or her with additional resources for disputing an MCO's decision. Fortunately, if the steps in this chapter are followed, very few disputes will ever reach this level.

Provider Responsibilities

As a network provider afforded many important rights, you must also be aware of your many responsibilities. In addition to the responsibilities of being an ethical provider of mental health services, BHN (2005) also lists several important responsibilities of providers working with managed care:

- Discussing any concerns you have
- Asking questions about eligibility, waiting periods, benefits, co-payments, and allowed number of visits
- Notifying the MCO of any concerns you have regarding coverage for your services
- Meeting all accessibility requirements
- Submitting outpatient treatment reports prior to the last authorized day
- Notifying the MCO if you are unable to accept new referrals and when you have reopened to new referrals
- Providing confidential and quality services
- Cooperating with all utilization management, quality assurance, and peer review programs

- Informing members of the costs of your services
- Abiding by your contract requirements
- Informing members of your duty to report child abuse and the threat of harm to self or others
- Taking corrective action on any issues identified through the complaint process
- Making appropriate referrals when needed

As you can see, the spirit of these responsibilities is that providers should look out for the best interest of their patients. One of the most important aspects is helping your patients navigate the managed care system.

Understanding Your Patient's Benefits

As mentioned previously, patients typically have an outpatient mental health benefit limit ranging from 20 to 60 vsits per year. Other patients will have an unlimited number of visits. Some patients will have a co-pay while others will have none. From your first meeting, you should take the time to explain these benefits and work collaboratively with your patient to develop a plan for managing the benefits. Keep in mind that MCOs offer a wide variety of benefit plans, so you cannot assume that every member of an MCO will have the same benefits as a member that you saw previously.

When appropriate, it is a good idea to help your patient understand other aspects of his or her mental health benefits. If inpatient services may be likely in the future, you should review your patient's inpatient benefits. Keep in mind that inpatient benefits can be very different from outpatient benefits. For example, you may have a patient with unlimited outpatient mental health visits with no co-pay, but an inpatient mental health benefit of only 30 mental health or substance abuse days per year and a $1,000 deductible. Discovering these benefits can help you and your patient prepare for future financial and treatment needs. Remember, the more information you can provide to the patient in a manner that can easily be understood, the better your patient will be able to navigate the managed care environment.

Summary Tips

- File your appeal as soon as you are sent written notification of an adverse decision you feel is unjust.
- If your appeal is denied, pursue another appeal at a higher level.

- For appeals involving cases you consider to be emergencies, request an expedited appeal.
- Make copies of all materials you submit to the MCO during the appeals process.
- Keep copies of all written denials and other documents from the MCO.
- The request for review of an administrative denial should also include a clear explanation of the circumstances, steps taken to avoid future occurrences, and the desired action from the MCO.
- When requesting a fair hearing, make sure to find out if the MCO's policies allow for legal representation and whether or not the MCO will be represented by an attorney.
- When requesting a fair hearing, be sure to read the documents explaining the fair hearing procedures.
- Before appealing, review your MCO's utilization and appeals procedures.
- Include only personal information that is relevant to your appeal.

CHAPTER EIGHT

Your Financial Relationship With Managed Care: Getting Paid

For most mental health providers, the purpose of working with managed care is to generate a lucrative revenue stream. To accomplish this, you will want to develop a rewarding financial relationship in which you are paid for your services in the timeliest manner possible. Thus you will need to understand the impact of third-party payment on providers. Since providers can be paid in several ways, you should also be familiar with the most common payment types. This chapter also provides strategies for obtaining payment for your services quicker and avoiding delays in processing of your claims.

The Impact of Third Party Payment

Managed care companies have become the so-called third party involved in health care delivery, with the other two parties being the patient and the provider delivering the services. The advent of MCOs and third-party payment more than half a century ago has altered the face of health care delivery, bringing about important changes that you as a provider should understand. Third-party health coverage from its earliest development enabled people to access health care when, where, and from whomever they needed it. By limiting barriers to access, this payment design is aimed at getting patients into care early and keeping them in care as long as necessary and with their provider of choice. The overall result of this system has been health care spending at unsustainable levels. As a result, over the years, managed care has developed payment strategies to help control the cost of health care. These strategies, however, have typically required the consumer or the provider to assume a greater financial burden for health care costs (Fendrick & Chernew, 2006). MCO strategies for controlling costs aimed at consumers include such things as co-payments, insurance deductibles, and coinsurance. Strategies aimed at providers include fee-for-service rates lower than providers charge, discounted fees, and other payment arrangements described later in this chapter.

In addition to criticisms of the increased cost to consumers and decreased revenue for providers, detractors of the third-party payment system also cite several other concerns. Since health insurance is often tied to employment by medium-sized to large employers, many citizens have been left without coverage. The involvement of a third-party payer also gives rise to concerns about confidentiality, particularly when health insurance contracts typically give third parties a right to access most if not all health-related information. It should also be noted that the third-party system is not viewed by MCOs as being without serious flaws. From the managed care perspective, serious concerns exist because health care is one of the few (and perhaps only) places where those receiving services do not have much or in some cases any responsibility for payment. Thus there is little incentive for the consumer to reduce unnecessary costs. This is why many of the MCO strategies developed to control costs have attempted to directly impact the wallets of consumers.

Another impact of the third-party payment system has been an increased oversight of providers. MCOs have the fiduciary responsibility to ensure that the services they are paying for are delivered at the highest clinical standards by properly trained and licensed professionals. To meet this responsibility, MCOs need to closely monitor the activities of providers to continually make sure that the highest quality of care is being delivered at a reasonable cost. This monitoring and oversight can also create stress for providers, who may view it as intrusive to their practice and their private relationship with patients. However, learning to deal with some level of oversight is part of working in the managed care environment.

Most providers and their patients have a pretty good understanding of the ways in which managed care can affect the care that is delivered. In most cases, third-party payment does not create much of an obstacle to care for patients or reimbursement for providers. As a provider, you must be aware not only of the impact of third-party payment but of the different payment types that are available and how they can impact your financial success.

Payment Types

You should be aware that MCOs offer various payment arrangements to providers. The common payment arrangements offered, including fee-for-service, discounted fee-for-service, capitation, contact capitation, and privileged provider compensation, vary by MCO. As a provider, you should understand of each of these payment arrangements in order to know which will work best for you.

Fee-for-Service

Under a fee-for-service arrangement, you as a provider agree to accept the MCO's rate of reimbursement for each service you provide. Rates are established by the MCO and typically differ by the type of service rendered, the type of provider rendering the service, the region in which the services are delivered, and the supply of providers available in that region. This payment arrangement is most beneficial for providers when the fee paid is acceptable and the MCO is able to generate a fair amount of referrals.

Discounted Fee-for-Service

A discounted arrangement is the same as the fee-for-service arrangement except that the reimbursement rate is typically lower. This arrangement is probably beneficial for providers only when the MCO is able to generate a high number of referrals.

Capitation

In a capitation arrangement, you as a provider are assigned a number of members. Typically those assigned will be a large group of members living in the geographic area where you practice. The members assigned to you will not all have mental health conditions. In fact, only a very small percentage will be seeking any treatment from you at all. Under this arrangement, the MCO pays you a fixed amount of money each month for each member assigned to you, regardless of how many or how few of these members you actually treat for mental health conditions.

It is expected that you will treat only a relatively small number of members. Therefore, the MCO will expect that you will be available to see these members as soon as they need you and for as long as they need you. This payment arrangement works best for providers when few of the assigned members require mental health services or at least few require intensive services. The care management under this arrangement is completely up to you as a provider, so you will have to balance the financial pressure to reduce the frequency of visits with the clinical necessity of providing appropriate care. What is important to remember about capitation arrangements is that you are at risk for losing money in that your reimbursement rate per session may fall well below what you normally receive for services if you have many members requiring many sessions. Providers in underserved areas such as rural communities and inner-city areas may be more likely to be offered this type of payment arrangement.

Contact Capitation

Contact capitation is a variation of capitation. In this payment system, which tends to be most appropriate for outpatient psychotherapy care, you as a provider are paid a fixed yearly fee at the time a patient assigned to you contacts you for an initial consultation for treatment. The fee is based on an average number of sessions utilized by MCO members each year. For example, you may receive $1,200 per year to manage each member that presents to your office. The care management of these members is left to you as a provider with little oversight from the MCO. If you are able to see most of these members for less than the average number of sessions, you will earn more money per session than if you need to see most members for more than the average. Most MCOs, however, will review the average number of visits that each patient received. The MCO will often modify the capitation upward for members found to require a much greater than average number of sessions. If you are considering accepting a contact capitation payment arrangement, make sure that you first find out if the MCO offers you any protection in the form of higher rates for members seen for many sessions above the average.

Privileged Provider Compensation

Some MCOs offer a unique compensation package to a few selected, privileged providers. These providers are clinicians considered by the MCO to have special qualifications, skills, or services required by the MCO, for which the MCO is willing to pay a higher than usual reimbursement rate for services provided. In the current managed care environment, privileged provider compensation may be offered to providers able to guarantee immediate access to care, particularly for patients just discharged from psychiatric hospitalization or who are at risk for future psychiatric hospitalization. Other providers offered this payment arrangement are

---

SPOTLIGHT ON

Capitation

Under most capitation arrangements, you will be financially at risk in that you could possibly have to provide a great deal of services, thus reducing your average fee per session. Before agreeing to capitation payment, you should ask the following questions:

- What is the overall average number of sessions per member seen, which the payment structure is based on?
- What is my personal average number of sessions per patient seen?
- Does the MCO have an average number of sessions per person seen in my geographical area?
- How many members will be assigned to me?
- What percentage of the MCO's membership utilize their outpatient mental health benefit?
- Is there a high rate of more serious mental illness requiring careful monitoring in my geographic area?
- Does the MCO offer any financial protection to me if I have to see certain patients for many more sessions than the average?
- If the MCO offers financial protection, how many sessions above average are needed before I become eligible for the extra reimbursement?
- Are community resources available that can be utilized to reduce the number of sessions a member will need with me?
- Do most of the members that would be assigned to me have an outpatient mental health benefit limit or are most eligible for unlimited appointments?
- How comfortable am I working within a short-term treatment model?

---

considered by the MCO to be experts in a particular field with an excellent reputation in the community. MCOs using this arrangement are willing to pay extra to be able to offer access to these providers to their members.

In addition to the payment arrangements described, some indemnity insurers, preferred provider organizations (PPOs), point-of-service (POS) plans, and health maintenance organizations (HMOs) offer an opportunity for providers to receive a bonus on top of their contracted payment arrangements. This opportunity is known as pay for performance. Pay for performance is still more commonly offered to medical providers but its popularity in the mental health arena is growing. Under pay for performance, an MCO will monitor the performance of all providers on a given measure (e.g., the percentage of members diagnosed with depression and started on antidepressant medication that are seen for at least three follow-up appointments within 3 months). Providers performing above a certain cutoff on the measure or providers performing within a given percentile as compared to their peers are identified and given additional compensation as a reward for their performance. It is therefore a good idea to review your contract, check your provider manual, read the newsletter, and speak with provider relations staff members to find out if the MCO offers pay for performance and to find out exactly what criteria will be used to judge provider performance.

Types of Insurance Coverage

It is helpful to understand the types of insurance coverage products that are commonly offered to consumers, as these products can impact the type of payment arrangements offered to you as a provider. The most common types of products available are indemnity coverage, PPO, POS, and HMO.

Indemnity Coverage

Indemnity coverage is a costly type of coverage for consumers. In exchange for the high cost, consumers typically have a choice of a very large number of providers. Plans providing indemnity coverage tend to pay providers according to the customary charges often set by a community of peers in the region in which the service is delivered. Additional payments may be made to selected mental health providers who offer a subspecialty that few others in the geographical area are able to offer.

- Choice of providers offered to members: high
- Reimbursement rate for providers: high
- Amount of MCO oversight: low

Preferred Provider Organizations

Preferred provider organizations are the most common type of managed care payment system and are very similar to indemnity plans. The PPO is also the fastest growing type of plan available to consumers, representing over half of total health plan enrollment (Gabel et al., 2003). In this type of payment arrangement, providers sign up to become part of a provider system offered to the MCO's members. Providers are listed in a book or on a Web site to which plan members have direct access. Depending on the rules of the MCO, a plan member may have direct access to listed providers without getting prior approval for their service. In exchange for becoming one of many participating providers in the PPO, the mental health professional agrees to accept the MCO's reimbursement rate. Although reimbursement rates in PPOs tend to be lower than in indemnity plans, oversight from the MCO is also low to moderate. In fact, some large managed care PPOs limit their services to network development and maintenance, which is often limited to simply the credentialing and recredentialing of providers.

- Choice of providers offered to members: high
- Reimbursement rate for providers: moderate
- Amount of MCO oversight: low to moderate

Point-of-Service Plan

The POS, a variation on the PPO plan, provides a comprehensive panel of participating providers from which the member may choose. If the member selects a participating provider from that panel, then the service is paid for in total by the MCO. However, if the plan member decides to see a nonparticipating provider, then the member will have to pay for a portion of the services, which may include both high deductibles and high co-pays. In fact, members seeing providers that are not part of the MCO's panel of providers will typically have to self-pay between 25% and 50% of the fees charged by the provider.

- Choice of providers offered to members: high
- Reimbursement rate for providers: moderate
- Amount of MCO oversight: moderate

Health Maintenance Organization

Members of HMOs trade provider choice and direct access to specialty providers (including behavioral health) for lower premiums (in many cases). Reimbursement rates for providers in HMO plans tend to be low compared to those for other types of products. HMOs also tend to have the greatest oversight of providers. The benefit for providers is that HMOs tend to be able to provide a greater number of patient referrals.

- Choice of providers offered to members: low to moderate
- Reimbursement rate for providers: low
- Amount of MCO oversight: high

Once you understand of the different payment types available, you will be in a better position to select an arrangement that works best for you and your practice.

Getting Paid Quicker

As a provider, you will receive payment for your services once you have fully completed and submitted a claim form. The CMS-1500, formerly known as the HCFA-1500, is the claim form used by most MCOs for outpatient services and includes a procedure code. The UB-92 is the claim form used by most MCOs for inpatient services and includes a revenue code. Many MCOs will not give these forms to providers. If your MCO does not make them available, you can obtain them at most office supply stores as they are standard in the industry. Most MCOs will also allow you to photocopy blank claim forms, but before doing this you should check with your MCO. You should also check with your MCO's provider relations department or provider manual for the correct address to which you should submit your claims.

Prior to submitting a claim, there are several steps you can take to decrease the time it takes to receive payment.

Step 1: Check Coverage

Membership coverage is highly volatile. A patient who was covered for outpatient mental health services at his or her last visit with you may no longer have coverage with that MCO at the current visit. Even if your session was previously authorized, if the member is no longer covered by the MCO, your claim will be denied. Submitting a claim for services rendered to a member who is no longer covered by the MCO is one of the most common reasons for denial of payment. As a result, you should check your patient's eligibility as often as possible. In fact, Community Behavioral HealthCare Network of Pennsylvania (2004) recommends that providers check member eligibility at least every 2 weeks. Typically, there are two ways in which you can check your patient's eligibility: online and via telephone.

Many MCOs now have online service available through their Web site that will allow you to check a member's eligibility as well as the authorization status after you register online as a provider. If this option is not available, you can simply call the MCO's provider relations department to find out your patient's eligibility.

Step 2: Check for Completeness

The second step you should take prior to submitting a claim is to check that the form was completed correctly. Remember, even simple, seemingly trivial information that is omitted from the form will result in rather lengthy delays in processing. The most common errors on submitted claim forms tend to be in the codes provided, specifically CPT codes, place-of-service codes, and ICD-9-CM (International Classification of Diseases, 9th Revision, Clinical Modification) codes. The following sections describe proper coding. However, you must keep in mind that codes may change over time and that you should check with your MCO to make sure that you are using the most up-to-date codes possible.

Current Procedural Terminology Codes

CPT codes represent the services provided by health care professionals. These codes inform the MCO of the type of service that was provided to the member. Table 8.1 is a nonexhaustive list and description of CPT codes commonly used by outpatient providers.

Keep in mind that these are only a few of the CPT codes available to providers. You should take the time to learn the CPT codes of the services that you will be performing for the MCO. If you have any questions regarding CPT codes, immediately call the provider relations department for clarification. Remember, the few minutes you spend on the phone obtaining clarification can save you weeks if not months waiting for your claim to be paid. Also keep in mind that codes can change over time, so it is a good idea to verify the codes that you are most likely to use.

Place-of-Service Codes

Place-of-service codes inform the MCO of the setting in which your service was delivered. It is important that your CPT codes and revenue codes be consistent with your place-of-service code. Keep in mind that codes change over time and that you must check with your MCO to make sure you are using the most up-to-date coding.

TABLE 8.1. Common CPT Codes

CPT Code	Description	Notes
90801	This code is used for the psychiatric diagnostic interview examination completed during the initial assessment. This assessment should include a history, mental status, disposition, and documentation of any collateral information. It may also include interpretation or ordering of laboratory or medical tests.	This code, often paid at a higher rate than a general session, may only be used for the initial session for the condition or suspected condition. It may be used again for the same member if the condition has been treated but then reoccurs and the member is seen for another initial session. Also, due to the nature of these sessions, the appropriate time frame for conducting the initial session would be in excess of 60 minutes. It is therefore a good idea to document in the medical record the length of this initial session.
90802	This code is used when evaluating children who do not have the ability to interact using ordinary verbal communication. This code can also apply to the initial assessment of adults who are unable to communicate using ordinary verbal communication.	When using this code, you should document in the medical record exactly what was used to overcome the communication deficits. For example, a provider might use a doll or toy to communicate with a child or a sign language interpreter to communicate with a deaf adult.
90804	This code is used for individual psychotherapy sessions lasting between 20 and 30 minutes.	Document the length of the session in the medical record. This code also specifies the use of insight-oriented, behavior modifying, or supportive techniques. Techniques used should be documented in the medical record.
90805	This code is used for individual psychotherapy sessions that include a medication evaluation	Document the length of the session in the medical record and document the psychotherapy techniques used in the

Code	Description	Notes
	...and medication management that last between 20 and 30 minutes	session (e.g., taught diaphragmatic breathing, conducted imaginal exposure).
90806	This code is used for individual psychotherapy sessions lasting between 45 and 50 minutes.	Document the length of the session in the medical record. Psychotherapy techniques used should also be documented in the medical record.
90807	This code is used for individual psychotherapy sessions that include a medication evaluation and medication management that last between 45 and 50 minutes.	Document the length of the session and the psychotherapy techniques in the medical record.
90846	This code is used for family therapy without the presence of the member who is the identified patient.	If the member who is the identified patient is present, use the 90847 code. Also, many MCOs, such as Value Options (2005), require family sessions to be at least 45 to 50 minutes long. This should be documented in the medical record.
90847	This code is used for family therapy when the member who is the identified patient is present.	Keep in mind that if the member who is the identified patient is not present, you would use the 90846 code. Also, many MCOs, such as Value Options (2005), require family sessions to be at least 45 to 50 minutes long. This should be documented in the medical record.
90862	This code is used for a medication check for an individual patient.	Be sure to document in the medical record that a medication check was performed.
99404	This code is used for EAP (Employee Assistance Program) sessions. Reimbursement is typically the same as for 90806.	Remember to use this code for EAP sessions.

ICD-9-CM Codes

A final common error on claim forms involves ICD-9-CM codes. These codes represent the diagnosis of the member being treated. Claims submitted with outdated or incomplete diagnostic codes will be denied. One common error resulting in incomplete diagnostic codes occurs when a provider omits the digits up to two decimal places. For example, a claim with an ICD-9-CM code of 300 for a diagnosis of anxiety disorder not otherwise specified may be denied and need to be resubmitted with an ICD-9-CM code of 300.00. Therefore, be sure you include the entire diagnostic code on all claims submitted. You should also keep in mind that many MCOs, such as Pacificare Behavioral Health (2005b), will not accept an ICD-9-CM code of 799.90, which is the code for diagnosis deferred.

Step 3: Submitting the Claim

Once you have verified your patient's eligibility and have made sure that you have completed the claim form correctly, it is time to submit the claim. Keep in mind that the faster you submit your claim, the faster you will receive payment. Not only is timely submission key to timely payment, it is also a requirement of most MCOs. Cigna Behavioral Health (2005), for example, reports that claims must be submitted within 60 days of the covered services being rendered. Claims submitted later than this are subject to denial.

MCOs will give you an address to mail your submitted claims to. Of course, before mailing a claim you should verify that you have the correct address. Luckily, mailing is not the only vehicle for claims submission. More and more MCOs are offering providers the opportunity to submit their claims electronically. If your MCO offers this option, it is strongly recommended that you submit your claims electronically rather than through the mail. There are several advantages to electronic (online) claims submission:

- Electronic claims submissions are almost always processed faster. In fact, Cigna Behavioral Health (2005) reports that all electronic claims that autoadjudicate are processed within 15 days.
- Electronic submission is usually free.
- Electronic submission is generally much more secure than mail-based submissions.
- Electronic submissions are more efficient with fewer errors than paper claims.
- Electronic submissions require less paper, labor, and postage expenses.
- You can usually track your claim online and find out as soon as its status has changed.

The process for utilizing Web-based electronic claims submission is usually rather simple, even if you are not very comfortable using a computer. While each MCO may have a different system, most MCOs will require some version of the following steps to gain access to their electronic, Web-based claims submission process:

1. Log onto the MCO's Web site.
2. Click on the icon for providers to submit claims.
3. Create a unique login and password to access the Web page.
4. Provide user account verification. These data can be used to verify you in case you forget your password in the future.
5. Provide the requested provider information (e.g., name, address, e-mail, etc.).

Generally speaking, after completing these steps you will be able to log onto the Web site, enter your user name and password, and then enter the system. Once in the system you will generally be able to submit your claims online and verify member eligibility. It is, however, recommended that you print copies of your online claims with the corresponding confirmation page for your personal records. Some systems also provide you with an e-mail account so that the MCO can e-mail you important messages. You may even have the option of e-mailing questions to the MCO rather than having to call and be placed on hold.

If the MCO does not offer Web-based submission of claims, or if you have simply elected to continue using paper-based claim submissions, there are several strategies you should employ to increase the timeliness of payment and reduce the need for resubmissions of your claims. Value Options New Mexico (2005) offers the following recommendations when submitting paper claims:

- Use black ink.
- Use original red-line claim forms.
- Use eight-digit dates. For example, if you provided a service on October 12, 2004, record the date as 10122004.
- Keep your print within the allotted boxes.
- Use uppercase letters.
- Avoid the use of dashes, slashes, circles, or other characters that could delay processing.
- If possible, type the claims.
- Consider using Courier 10 font or above.
- Do not fold or staple anything to the claim.
- Provide additional comments on a separate piece of paper.

- Include your patient's date of birth.
- Whenever possible, use "signature on file," assuming that the MCO does have your signature on file already.

Common Pitfalls That Delay Payment

After you have verified your patient's eligibility, checked the accuracy of your coding, and submitted your claims in a timely manner, there are still a few pitfalls that can delay your claims processing and payment that you should avoid:

- Making handwritten corrections
- Using correction fluid to make changes to claims
- Omitting your provider identification number, which identifies you as a contracted provider
- Omitting your vendor identification number, which identifies the location where your service was rendered
- Omitting your federal tax identification number
- Submitting a claim for a date of service that is prior to or after the authorized benefit period
- Billing for an unauthorized service
- Billing for a service delivered after a member terminated his or her insurance coverage
- Billing for a service delivered after the member's benefits have been exhausted
- Submitting a claim as a provider other than the provider who was authorized to give services (e.g., authorization for outpatient therapy was given for a social worker but the services were provided by a psychologist)

In addition to these pitfalls, avoid submitting your claims late. Keep in mind that you may submit a claim on time, but if it gets lost in the mail or by the MCO it will be considered late and therefore subject to denial. For this reason, it is a good practice to periodically check the status of your claim either online or by telephone. Many MCOs, including Cigna Behavioral Health (2005) will allow you to submit proof of timely filing of a claim that was denied for lateness. An account ledger showing the original date that you submitted the claim will often be accepted in good faith. It is therefore worth the extra step of logging your claim submissions in a personal ledger in case you are ever confronted with this problem. Of course, electronic submission of claims allows you to avoid this altogether as you get immediate confirmation that the claim was received and you are able to track the processing online.

Once you have completed and submitted your claim, how long should you expect to wait before you receive payment? Although the wait time can vary, most MCOs will process payment of clean, paper-based claims (claims completely free of errors) within 30 days (Cigna Behavioral Health, 2005; Community Behavioral HealthCare Network of Pennsylvania, 2004). It is important to know how long it takes your MCO to process clean claims so that you will know how long to wait before looking for a missing payment. One final pitfall that many providers fall into involves duplicate billing. In this scenario, a provider who has not yet received payment will submit an additional claim for the same service during the processing time hoping that the second claim submitted will be paid. This can create problems as both claims could mistakenly be paid. If the provider does not realize this, or does realize it yet fails to return one of the payments, he or she could be guilty of abuse or fraud. Submitting duplicate claims within a short time may also violate the terms of your provider contract. For example, Cigna Behavioral Health (2005) states that participating providers agree to refrain from duplicate billing within 30 days of submitting a bill for covered services. Unless otherwise instructed by your MCO, it is always preferable to check the status of your claim online or by calling the provider relations department rather than sending duplicate bills, particularly given that many MCO's now have automated telephone systems that can track your claim and are accessible 24 hours a day.

By following the recommendations presented in this section, you can markedly reduce the time it takes to receive payment for your services. You can also avoid having to spend precious time and energy fixing and resubmitting previously submitted claims due to minor errors.

Summary Tips

- Find out exactly what type of payment arrangements are offered by your MCO.
- If you are entering into any type of capitation arrangement, find out if the MCO will offer any financial protection for members that need to be seen well above the average number of sessions.
- Find out if your MCO offers pay for performance.
- If pay for performance is offered, find out what measures are used to rate providers.
- Submit all claims in a timely manner.

- Do not cross out or use correction fluid on submitted claims.
- Frequently verify your patient's coverage and benefit limitations.
- If available, use electronic submission of claims rather than submitting paper claims.
- Double-check that all codes are correct prior to submitting your claims.
- Keep a personal ledger of submitted claims.
- Use eight digits to record the dates on claims.
- Find out how long your MCO takes to process clean claims. If you have not received payment for a clean claim within that time, you should begin making inquiries to find out why.

CHAPTER NINE

Building Your Practice With Managed Care

If you joined a managed care network, chances are you did so to build your practice in order to ultimately increase your income. However, simply being on an MCO's list of providers is unlikely to generate a large volume of referrals unless you happen to be located in an area with few other providers or have a specialty that few providers in your area can offer. Since these scenarios are unlikely, you should develop strategies for generating more referrals from the MCO. This chapter will provide you with strategies for increasing your appeal to the MCO by demonstrating quality. The strategies will allow you to demonstrate quality in a way that the MCO will recognize. This chapter details how to demonstrate success on commonly used quality measures, how to succeed on provider profiling, how to use clinical practice guidelines to your advantage, and how to utilize outcome measures.

Demonstrating Quality

All providers want to provide high-quality treatment to their patients. MCOs also want to make sure that their members are receiving treatment that meets the highest standards. The questions then become: What is quality care? And how can it be demonstrated? The answer to these questions in many respects depends upon who is asking them. To a provider, quality treatment might mean getting to a point where a patient with posttraumatic stress disorder is finally able to openly discuss traumatic experiences in session, or helping a patient with panic disorder begin to travel unaccompanied once again, or it might mean getting to a point where a patient no longer has panic attacks. While there are many different possible ways in which quality treatment can be operationalized for each individual patient, MCOs must take a different perspective when it comes to demonstrating quality. While providers often view the quality of treatment on a case-by-case or condition-by-condition basis, MCOs must define quality in a way that is applicable to a whole network of providers and often across many different conditions and patients.

So how do MCOs define quality? Many providers believe that MCOs are interested in having providers get their members functioning at the level they were at just prior to requiring treatment as fast as possible with as few sessions as possible. However, most MCOs do not measure quality in terms of how few sessions a provider utilizes. Instead, most MCOs have a few clearly defined quality indicators that they use to judge quality. While these indicators vary, any MCO accredited by NCQA or that is planning to apply for accreditation from NCQA needs to report key behavioral health indicators or measures. In addition, MCOs not planning to pursue NCQA accreditation often choose to adopt the same measures because they are quickly becoming a standard in the industry and because they reflect guidelines for health care quality developed by the Agency for Health Care Research and Quality (NCQA, 2004).

Success on these measures is critical for achieving and maintaining NCQA accreditation, the importance of which cannot be overstated. As you are aware, accreditation is critical in marketing an MCO to potential employer groups who purchase health insurance for their employees. Loss of accreditation or poor performance can result in a reduction in membership, revenue, and serious difficulties marketing that MCO to new customers. Because these measures are so important, MCOs typically use them to judge the quality of its network providers. For this reason, if you are interested in expanding your practice through managed care, you should become very familiar with NCQA's behavioral health standards, because chances are your MCO will be very interested in your performance on them. Therefore, to get recognized as a valuable provider, you will need to demonstrate success on these measures of quality.

Documenting Success on Quality Measures

NCQA has developed a set of standardized performance measures that are used to rate MCOs. The set of standards, known as HEDIS (Health Plan Employer Data

TABLE 9.1. **Behavioral Health Measures**

Measure	*Components*
Follow-up after psychiatric hospitalization	7-day follow-up 30-day follow-up
Antidepressant medication management	Optimal contacts Acute-phase treatment Continuous-phase treatment
Alcohol and other drug dependence	Initiation Engagement
Follow-up for children prescribed ADHD medicine	Initiation Phase Continuous Phase

Information Set), contain measures in all areas of health care delivery. The behavioral health measures that you should become familiar with are listed in Table 9.1. Each of these measures is described in more detail below along with the reasons they are important to MCOs. The definition of each measure is paraphrased because it is the spirit of the measure that is most important for providers to understand as opposed to the intricacies of the specifications. For the exact, highly detailed definition, you can visit NCQA's Web site (www.ncqa.org). Also, keep in mind that all of these measures are inherently important to MCOs simply by virtue of the fact that they are HEDIS measures. Recent trends on the measures are also presented along with strategies that you can employ to achieve success on them. Knowing and understanding these measures is the key to speaking the language of managed care. This understanding will allow you to flourish within the managed care environment and will help ensure that your MCO will be motivated to send referrals to you as you demonstrate success on the measures that matter the most to them.

Follow-up After Hospitalization for Mental Illness

This standard measures the percentage of members age 6 and older that receive an ambulatory (outpatient) follow-up visit after being discharged following inpatient treatment for a mental health disorder. It is reported in terms of percentage seen for follow-up within 7 days and within 30 days.

Importance of the Measure to MCOs
This measure is important because appropriate follow-up care helps to reduce the risk of repeat hospitalizations for some people and identifies those in need of

further hospitalization before they reach a mental health or medical crisis (Boydell, Malcolmson, & Sikerbol, 1991). The use of appropriate mental health services also tends to decrease inappropriate use of medical services, resulting in overall health savings.

Trends

According to NCQA (2004), reporting plans have been slow to improve performance over time on this measure. In fact, on average only slightly more than half of the commercial insurance members meeting criteria for the 7-day measure were seen for follow-up within 7 days. For Medicaid and Medicare members, the rate was less than 39%. MCOs have worked hard to try to improve performance on this measure with little success. Therefore any provider in an MCO's network demonstrating success on this measure will be highly valued. Once identified, that therapist is likely to receive additional referrals.

Strategies for Demonstrating Success on This Measure

- Have a policy that you will see any member discharged from the hospital within 24 hours (or any similar time frame that you can reasonably adhere to) and inform your MCO of that policy. Make sure that the provider relations department is aware that you give post–hospital discharge patients the highest priority and that no matter what your general availability you will do whatever it takes to ensure that any post–hospital discharge patient is given an appointment within 24 hours. You may even be able to negotiate a higher rate for these services if you agree to grant these members immediate access.
- Be tenacious. One of the main reasons MCOs have had difficulty improving performance on this measure is not because post–hospital discharge patients are not given timely appointments—it is because many of these patients do not show up for these appointments. Therefore, do everything possible to ensure that members discharged from the hospital are seen as soon as possible.
  - When a post-hospital member calls for an appointment, be sure to get his or her telephone number, cell phone number, address, and any other contact information that can help you reach him or her if the appointment is missed. Keep in mind that the MCO's contact information may not be up to date. Some of these members may not currently have stable living situations, so being able to reach them in the future is vitally.
  - Give an appointment within 24 hours. This way, if the appointment is broken you will still have time to see the member in time for success on this measure. Early contact will also facilitate greater continuity of care, which is of course critical to the success of treatment (Boydell et al., 1991).

- Be sure to call and remind the member about the appointment. Even if you spoke to the member yesterday and gave an appointment for today, call today and remind that member of the appointment time and location.
- Be sure the member knows exactly where you are located and has the means to get to the appointment. Any difficulty finding your office can easily result in a broken appointment.
- If the member cannot travel to the appointment, call the MCO and let them know that this member meets criteria for this measure and is unable to get to the appointment. The MCO may be able to provide transportation in order to have success on the measure. Even if this is not possible, your call will serve to remind the MCO that you are aware of these measures and working hard to achieve success.
- If the appointment is broken, call the member immediately to reschedule. If you are unable to reach the member initially, continue trying to reschedule. If calling fails, try sending a timely outreach letter as well. You may also consider contacting the MCO to find out if additional contact information is available.

Antidepressant Medication Management: Effective Acute-Phase Treatment

This standard measures the percentage of an MCO's eligible members who remained on an antidepressant medication for a new episode of depression (e.g., major depression, dysthymia) during the 12-week acute treatment phase.

Importance of the Measure to MCOs
This measure is important because a very high percentage of patients initiating antidepressant medication terminate the medication on their own or do not take it as prescribed (Unutzer, Katon, & Callahan, 2002; Wells, Sherbourne, & Schoenbaum, 2000). MCOs realize that inadequate medication or premature termination of medication places a member at an increased risk of depression relapse or a general worsening of symptoms (Bull, Hu, & Hunkeler, 2002). It also represents wasted expense as the MCO paid for the medication that is not being taken appropriately (Weilberg, Stafford, O'Leary, Meigs, & Finkelstein, 2004).

Trends
According to NCQA (2004), results on this measure have shown a lack of overall improvement, with current results similar to those reported in 1999. In fact, NCQA (2004) reported that only approximately 60% of commercial insurance members, 53% of Medicare members, and 46% of Medicaid members achieved success on

this measure. Therefore, any provider demonstrating success on this measure will be highly attractive to an MCO.

Strategies for Demonstrating Success on This Measure
- Discuss the importance of proper medication adherence with all members you see who are taking antidepressant medication.
- Document this discussion in the treatment record. This will look very good to any future reviewer from an MCO who may audit the chart. It is also good clinical practice and part of quality depression care.
- If you are not the prescribing physician, obtain the member's consent to collaborate with the prescribing physician, whether he or she is a psychiatrist, PCP, or any other type of prescriber. A therapist's input on medication adherence and effect of medication is often helpful in the medication process and can lead to improved adherence (Beck, 2001; Coyne, Thompson, Klinkman, & Neese, 2002; Kaintz, 2002; Kolbasovsky, Reich, Romano, & Jaramillo, 2005; McDaniel, Belar, Schroeder, Hargrove, & Freeman, 2002). Collaboration can also address progress toward success on the measure.
- Provide members with educational handouts about depression and proper medication adherence. Handouts on this topic can be found on the MacArthur Initiative on Depression in Primary Care Web site (www.depression-primarycare.org). Be sure to document in the medical record that you provided educational materials.
- See members newly started on antidepressant medication frequently, particularly in the beginning of treatment, to monitor side effects, adherence, and progress.
- Include medication adherence as part of your treatment plan. This will reinforce the importance of proper medication adherence to the member you are working with and it will demonstrate to the MCO that you are clearly working toward success on this measure.
- Discuss all member concerns and questions about antidepressant medication.
- Inform members starting on antidepressant medication that while antidepressants are not typically taken for life, it is recommended that most people remain on the medication for at least 6 months, and that you, the member, and the prescribing physician will work together to decide when is the right time to discontinue the medication (Lin, Von Korff, & Katon, 1995; NCQA, 2004).
- There is some evidence that PCPs may tend to keep patients at antidepressant dosages lower than what is needed to achieve a full therapeutic effect (Finley et al., 2003; U.S. Department of Health and Human Services, 1993). Collaborating with PCPs (or other prescribing physicians) and providing feedback

about progress, adherence, and symptoms may help to improve the medication care provided (Kolbasovsky et al., 2005).

Antidepressant Medication Management: Effective Continuation-Phase Treatment

This standard measures the percentage of an MCO's eligible members who remained on an antidepressant medication continuously for 6 months following an initial diagnosis of depression and treatment with an antidepressant medication.

Importance of the Measure to MCOs

This measure is important because a very high percentage of patients initiating antidepressant medication terminate the medication prior to the minimum recommended standard of 6 months (Lin et al., 1995; NCQA, 2004). MCOs realize that inadequate medication or premature termination of medication places a member at an increased risk of depression relapse or a general worsening of symptoms (Bull et al., 2002). It also represents wasted expense as the MCO paid for the medication, which is not being taken appropriately and therefore is very unlikely to have a significant positive effect on symptoms (Weilburg et al., 2004).

Trends

According to NCQA (2004), results on this measure have shown a lack of overall improvement, with current results similar to those reported in 1999. In fact, NCQA reported that only approximately 44% of commercial insurance members, 39% of Medicare members, and 29% of Medicaid members achieved success on this measure. Therefore, any provider demonstrating success on this measure will be highly attractive to an MCO.

Strategies for Demonstrating Success on This Measure

- All of the strategies listed for effective acute-phase treatment also apply to this measure.
- Continue to review medication adherence and document the review in the record for 6 months (and beyond).

Antidepressant Medication Management: Optimal Practitioner Contacts

This standard measures the percentage of an MCO's eligible members who received at least three follow-up visits with a prescribing physician or mental health provider in the 12-week acute treatment phase after a new diagnosis of depression and a prescription of an antidepressant medication. At least one of these follow-up visits must be with the prescribing physician.

Importance of the Measure to MCOs

This measure is important because of the high cost of major depression, the leading cause of disability in the United States (Conti & Burton, 1994).

Trends

According to NCQA (2004), results on this measure have shown a lack of overall improvement, with current results similar to those reported in 1999. In fact, NCQA reported that only approximately 20% of commercial insurance members, 11% of Medicare members, and 18% of Medicaid members achieved success on this measure. The lack of improvement in the antidepressant medication measures has led Scholle (2005) to conclude that there is room for much improvement in the HEDIS rates for depression. Therefore, any provider demonstrating success on this measure will be highly attractive to an MCO.

Strategies for Demonstrating Success on This Measure

- Be sure to identify all patients you see who meet criteria for this measure.
- Upon identification, inform your patient about the importance of proper follow-up with you and the prescribing physician.
- Provide education on antidepressant medication and answer any and all questions.
- Make sure that your patient has an appointment with the prescribing physician within 2 to 4 weeks of starting the antidepressant medication.
- Follow up to make sure the appointment was kept.
- Schedule follow-up appointments in a very timely fashion.
- Be sure to get updated contact information and multiple contact numbers if possible to help get the patient back into care after a canceled or broken appointment.
- If you have difficulty contacting the patient to reschedule, consider contacting the MCO and explaining that you are working with a member who meets criteria for the measure but has been unreachable. Ask if they have other contact information. It is a long shot that they will have better information than you, but this will also serve to remind the MCO of your diligence and the quality of care provided, particularly to members meeting criteria for this very important measure.

SPOTLIGHT ON

Identifying Patients Who Meet Criteria for the Measure

Although the antidepressant medication management measures are designed to monitor patients started on medication for a new episode of depression, anyone who has not been on any antidepressant medication for 3
months and has had no diagnosis submitted on a claim in the previous 4
months is considered to have a new episode. Therefore, you should be
aware that you may treat a patient on and off for a long time as he or she
drops in and out of care. This type of patient with a thick chart that you
may know for many years may meet criteria for the antidepressant medication management measures for a new episode of depression upon dropping
back into care and restarting antidepressant medication, even though to you
they do not seem like a new case at all. These are precisely the type of patients who often fail to get identified and perform worse on the medication
management measures. For this reason, make sure that you identify not
only your newly depressed patients started on medication but your returning or long-term patients as well.

- Incorporate attendance at the specified follow-up appointments and proper
  medication adherence into your treatment plan.
- If you are not the prescribing physician, get informed consent to consult with
  the prescribing physician so that you and the physician can work together to
  provide care and encourage adherence to all aspects of the treatment plan.

Initiation of Alcohol and Other Drug Dependence Treatment

This standard measures the percentage of adults diagnosed with alcohol and other
drug (AOD) dependence who initiate treatment through an inpatient admission or
through outpatient services for AOD abuse or dependence who have any additional AOD services within 14 days.

Importance of the Measure to MCOs
This measure is important because over 16 million Americans aged 12 or older are
dependent on or abuse alcohol or illicit drugs (SAMHSA, 2001). On top of the

high need for treatment, MCOs are aware that untreated alcohol- or drug-dependent persons use health care and incur costs at a rate about twice that of their age and gender cohorts (Holder, 1998) and once substance abuse treatment begins, total health care utilization and costs begin to drop, reaching a level that is lower than pretreatment costs after a 2- to 4-year period (Holder, 1998). In addition, individuals completing more days of treatment typically show more improvement than those leaving care prematurely (McLellan, 1997).

Trends
This is a new measure that was first reported in 2005. Results from the first year of reporting indicate that members with commercial, Medicare, and Medicaid insurance coverage achieve success on the initiation measure in 45.9%, 54.7%, and 45.7% of substance abuse cases meeting criteria for this measure, respectively (NCQA, 2005).

Strategies for Demonstrating Success on This Measure
- Realize that you should take responsibility for seeing any member with a substance abuse diagnosis for another session within 14 days. Knowing this standard will also make it easier for you to get future sessions approved.
- When requesting authorization for sessions, be sure to inform the MCO that the member for whom the sessions are requested meets criteria for this measure.
- When you diagnose a substance abuse disorder, be sure to set a follow-up appointment within 1 week, provide sufficient time to reschedule, if necessary, and still make the 2-week time period.
- Substance-abusing patients often break appointments. By scheduling a follow-up appointment early, you will have an opportunity to reschedule a missed appointment and still make the 14-day deadline for the measure.
- When you set up a follow-up appointment, be sure to get as many different contact numbers as possible before the patient leaves your office. Do not rely on information provided by the MCO as it may be out of date. The more contact information you have, the better your chance of rescheduling the appointment and having success on the measure.
- If you refer out for substance abuse treatment, make sure that your patient has an appointment with the referred provider within 1 week. If the facility does not offer an appointment to your patient within that time frame, call the MCO with the member in your office and explain that your patient meets criteria for the HEDIS measure and needs to be seen within a week. This serves two purposes: (1) the MCO will likely put pressure on the provider to get the

member seen quickly, thus improving the continuity of care provided to the member; and (2) it demonstrates to the MCO that you are not only aware of the measure, you are taking active steps to promote success on the measure.

- If you refer out for substance abuse treatment and are unable to get a timely appointment with a substance abuse provider, consider seeing the patient one more time (within the 14 days) while he or she is waiting for an appointment. This will allow for further evaluation, will improve continuity for the member, and can lead to success on the measure.

- Inform the MCO that it is your policy that anyone diagnosed with a substance abuse disorder be seen for a follow-up appointment within 1 week.

Engagement of AOD Dependence Treatment

This standard measures the percentage of adults diagnosed with AOD dependence that are seen for an additional two visits within 30 days after the initiation of AOD treatment (the initial session is when they were first diagnosed with AOD dependence).

Importance of the Measure to MCOs

This measure is important because more than half of all patients with AOD disorders leave treatment prematurely (Batten, Prottas, & Horgan, 1992) despite the fact that the frequency and intensity of engagement have been shown to be important variables in treatment outcomes and for reducing drug related illnesses (McLellan et al., 1997). In addition to health problems and costs associated with substance abuse, MCOs are also concerned because workers who use illicit drugs are more likely to change employers (which could mean a change of insurance), miss work due to illness or injury, or skip work more often than those who do not use illicit drugs (Substance Abuse Mental Health Services Administration, 2001). Keep in mind that missed work translates into increased costs for the employer groups contracted with the MCO. This is obviously an important concern for employers, which makes it an important concern for any MCO wishing to sell itself to employers.

Trends

This is a new measure that was first reported in 2005. The success rate for engagement is markedly lower than for initiation, with only 15.5%, 7.0%, and 12.0% of commercial, Medicare, and Medicaid members achieving successful treatment engagement, respectively (NCQA, 2005b). Clearly there is great room for improvement on this measure.

Strategies for Demonstrating Success on This Measure
- The strategies proposed for the initiation of AOD treatment measure are applicable for this measure.
- When you diagnose a member with substance abuse, try to schedule two timely follow-up sessions at the initial meeting. You can also inform the MCO when requesting authorization that this member meets criteria for the measure. This should speed the authorization process (if that is an issue).
- Stress the importance of treatment engagement in your clinical work. Do not forget to document this discussion in your notes, as this represents good clinical work and will look very favorable to the MCO.

Follow-up Care for Children Prescribed ADHD Medication: Initiation Phase

This standard measures the percentage of children (aged 6–12) newly prescribed ADHD medication who have a follow-up visit within 30 days of the drug being dispensed. This measure is currently in effect.

Importance of the Measure to MCOs
This measure is important because ADHD is highly prevalent and highly persistent, and there has been a sevenfold increase in prescriptions for stimulant medications during the past decade (American Academy of Pediatrics, 2000).

Trends
This measure is new, thus no trends are available.

Strategies for Success on This Measure
- Educate the parents of any child with ADHD that it is very important to have a follow-up visit within 2 weeks of starting a medication for ADHD and document this discussion in the medical record.
- If you are the prescribing physician, make sure that the child has a scheduled follow-up appointment.
- If you are not the prescribing physician, make sure the child has a follow-up appointment scheduled with the prescribing physician. If the child does not, help the family to set up an appointment with the prescribing provider.
- If you are not the prescribing physician, obtain a signed consent to collaborate with the prescribing physician. This can greatly improve the care provided and facilitate adherence to treatment appointments.

Follow-up Care for Children Prescribed ADHD Medication: Continuous and Maintenance Phases

This standard measures the percentage of children (aged 6–12) who remain on ADHD medication who have at least two additional follow-up visits within 9 months of the initiation visit.

Importance of the Measure to MCOs

This measure is important because regular visits and monitoring of medication and symptoms are an important aspect of treatment (American Academy of Pediatrics, 2000).

Trends

This measure is new, thus no trends are available.

Strategies for Demonstrating Success on This Measure

- The strategies listed for the initiation phase are applicable for this measure as well.
- Educate the parents of any child with ADHD that it is very important to have at least two follow-up visits within a few months (9 at the most) of the initiation phase follow-up and document this discussion.
- Be involved in facilitating the follow-up appointments.
- Incorporate attending follow-up sessions into your treatment plan. This reinforces the importance of follow-up to the family and reminds the MCO that you are diligently working toward success on this measure.

While it may seem tedious and somewhat repetitive to learn about each of these measures, knowing them is the key to understanding the motivation of MCOs and to speaking the language of managed care. You may be surprised to find out just how accommodating MCOs will be when you are able to identify members meeting criteria for these measures and to provide high-quality care to those members.

A provider familiar with these measures can speak to an MCO in a language that will be heard. While knowing these measures is not a secret password to get approval for services, it will help speed the process of approval when needed. It should be remembered that these measures are critical to all MCOs involved with NCQA credentialing. Obviously, an MCO that is not planning to pursue credentialing may be less interested in these measures. However, NCQA selected these measures because they are considered a minimum standard of care. For this reason it is a good idea for providers to be familiar with these measures and to perform well on them in order to provide high-quality care. Providers should keep in mind that credentialed MCOs as well as many MCOs not credentialed by NCQA are very likely to use these measures in order to conduct what is known as provider profiling.

Provider Profiling

Essentially, provider profiling is done by MCOs to measure the effectiveness (and thus desirability) of providers. Administrative data are used to give a rating on a particular measure or measures to each provider in the MCO's network. An individual provider is then compared to his or her peers based on the measure. While this may be relatively new for some MCOs, others, such as Foundation Health PsychCare, have done this since at least the mid-1990s (Hiatt & Hargrave, 1995). In many cases, MCOs will use one (or more) of the eight HEDIS measures listed above. For example, Value Options New Mexico (2005) lists performance standards for providers. Included in this list are discharge follow-up (7- and 30-day) and behavioral health HEDIS measures.

An MCO reviewing its providers' performance will look to refer more of its members to the providers demonstrating the greatest success on the quality measures. Thus, if you are looking to build your practice with managed care, it is imperative that you understand these measures and work to improve outcomes on them. By achieving success on the measures and therefore success during provider profiling, you may be placed on what is known as a preferred provider list. Preferred providers are often given special benefits and receive many more referrals from the MCO than those providers who are not on the list. In addition to the eight HEDIS measures, or in lieu of those measures, some MCOs will use their own measures to identify quality in its network. These measures can often be found in the MCO's clinical practice guidelines or in the provider relations manual. Additional, non-HEDIS measures often used by MCOs to measure the performance of its providers include (but are not limited to):

• Accessibility, particularly to patients recently discharged from a psychiatric hospitalization
• Evidence of communication with your patients' PCPs
• Member satisfaction with your services

- Psychiatric hospitalization readmission rates
- Compliance with MCO protocols

Clinical Practice Guidelines

The concept of clinical practice guidelines has been well established in the medical community for many years. They are now also becoming more and more standard in the field of mental health as well. Most if not all MCOs have developed clinical practice guidelines for the treatment of at least some behavioral health conditions, most often chronic conditions such as depression, ADHD, and substance abuse. MCO adoption of clinical practice guidelines is due in part to an effort to ensure a certain minimum level of care and because NCQA has determined that MCOs need to create, monitor, and revise (at least every 2 years) clinical practice guidelines. Because MCOs need to monitor these guidelines, most will include a measure within the guideline that the MCO can track using administrative data.

In some cases MCOs adopt already established clinical practice guidelines created by professional organizations such as the American Psychiatric Association (2002c) or they may choose to create their own clinical practice guidelines. For example, Magellan Health Services' (2004) provider manual contains each of its clinical practice guidelines. Magellan chose to create its own clinical practice guidelines for the treatment of adults with substance abuse disorders. In this guideline, it states that maintenance and recovery phase follow-up should occur at least every 3 months for 12 months' duration. Evidence of a maintenance plan and an assessment of functioning for alcohol abusers should also occur. With these statements, Magellan set minimum criteria for quality care. It is easy to see how Magellan could, if it so chose, identify members in the maintenance or recovery phases and monitor the percentage of members seen for the recommended sessions. This could then be used to rate providers.

Clinical practice guidelines are also a vehicle for MCOs to inform you of exactly what is expected of you when treating their members. Despite the importance of this, many providers do not bother to even read them. As a provider, you should familiarize yourself with the clinical practice guidelines of each MCO with which you are contracted. As you read the guidelines, look for recommendations that could be used to monitor performance since you now know that MCOs need to monitor their guidelines. As you read the guidelines with an eye toward possible measures the MCO may use for monitoring, you will likely notice that many of these guidelines incorporate standards set by NCQA with its HEDIS measures. For example, Harvard Pilgrim Health Care (2005) states that at least every 2 years it will select at least one specific indicator from its clinical practice guidelines and monitor activities related to that indicator. It goes on to state that the HEDIS anti-depressant measure will comprise at least part of the scheduled monitoring.

Clearly, monitoring the quality of care delivered by providers through the use of administratively identified measures has become commonplace for MCOs, with HEDIS measures being the most commonly used. You may have noticed that most of the measures presented have been process measures focused on number and timeliness of visits or adherence to treatment protocol as opposed to outcome measures focused on a decrease in symptom severity or improvement in function-ing. However, with so much emphasis now being placed on monitoring, it should come as no surprise that many MCOs are increasingly starting to utilize outcome measures in their monitoring of providers.

Outcome Measures

More and more MCOs are expecting providers to be accountable and to show tan-gible results of their work (Cohen, 2003; Zur, 1999). While the use of outcome measures is certainly less common than the use of process measures in monitor-ing performance, more and more MCOs are incorporating the use of outcome measurement. One company that has incorporated many outcome measures into its relationship with providers is Pacificare Behavioral Health with its ALERT sys-tem (ALgorithms for Effective Reporting and Treatment). Because this system has become well known in the managed care industry and because similar systems may be adopted by other MCOs in the near future, we provide a brief description of the ALERT system.

According to Pacificare Behavioral Health (2005b), ALERT is an outcomes man-agement system used to analyze change based on member self-report and assess-ment in combination with provider-reported data, which monitors data throughout a treatment episode while also comparing actual change to expected change. The ALERT system uses the Life Status Questionnaire (LSQ) for adults and the Youth Life Status Questionnaire (YLSQ) for children and teens, which are given repeat-edly throughout treatment. The ALERT system allows Pacificare to predict the ex-pected change scores (improvement) for each member in treatment and to identify members for whom the expected change is not yet occurring. The ALERT system is also used to identify the 10% of cases at the highest risk for poor outcomes. The ALERT system has determined that these cases are at high risk for dropping out of treatment. ALERT has also shown that when these members are maintained in treatment, significant improvements are often seen. Thus, steps are taken by Pacificare to promote adherence to treatment for these identified high-risk members.

The ALERT system also compares member response to provider report of symptoms, particularly in the areas of suicidal ideation and substance abuse. If a member reports having suicidal ideation "frequently" or "almost always" and the provider reports that he or she believed that the member does not have suicidal ideation, the ALERT system identifies this as nonconcordant responses, and the provider is sent a letter informing him or her of the discrepancy. Pacificare reported that upon starting this program in 2001, in 50% of the cases in which a member reported a high frequency of suicidal ideation, the provider assessed that there was no suicidal ideation (Beaudin et al., 2004; Brown, Jones, Betts, & Wu, 2003), thus further underscoring the importance of doing repeated, thorough suicide assessments in all cases. The same process is in place for identifying substance abuse. Similarly, the ALERT system has found that clinicians frequently underestimate the severity of members' substance use, thus underscoring the importance of conducting repeated, thorough substance abuse assessments. In addition to identifying at-risk cases and predicting outcomes, ALERT is used to identify providers who consistently achieve treatment progress beyond what is predicted by the system. These providers are identified and given a financial bonus as part of the Honors4Outcomes program (Beaudin, 2005; Jones, 2005).

While every MCO may not be systematically monitoring outcome measures for all providers, which can be a very costly and time-consuming proposition, most MCOs appreciate when providers incorporate outcome measures into their clinical work. There are several reasons to utilize outcome measures when working with managed care. As previously discussed, treatment plans should contain goals that are observable and measurable. Incorporating a questionnaire-based outcome measure into your goals is one way of ensuring a measurable goal. Using a questionnaire to track symptoms also allows you to demonstrate improvement and quality of care, which is of course desirable to an MCO. In addition, if your patient's symptoms worsen, having documentation of this on a measure will help you to make the case for the medical necessity of additional sessions. Finally, monitoring progress throughout treatment keeps you better informed and allows you to better tailor your treatment to the needs of your patient.

The outcome measures chosen to be used in treatment should be valid and reliable measures that best suit your needs and the needs of your patient. When working with MCOs, it is a good idea to select measures that are also well known. The following is a list of well-known, valid, and reliable measures often used in treatment for several different conditions commonly seen by outpatient providers. Keep in mind that this is by no means an exhaustive list and that many other good measures are available:

- **Patient Health Qusestionnaire–9** (PHQ-9; Spitzer, Kroenke, & Williams, 1999): The PHQ-9 is a nine-item depression assessment with items that correspond to the *DSM-IV* criteria for major depression.
- **Patient Health Questionnaire–15** (PHQ-15; Kroenke, Spitzer, & Williams, 2002): The PHQ-15 is a 15-item assessment of the severity of somatic symptoms.
- **PTSD Checklist–Civilian Version** (PCL-C; Weathers, Huska, & Keane, 1991): The PCL-C is a 17-item assessment tool for PTSD to be used with the civilian (as opposed to military) population. The items correspond with *DSM-IV* criteria for PTSD.
- **Alcohol Use Disorders Identification Test** (AUDIT; Babor, Higgins-Biddle, Saunders, & Monteiro, 2001): The AUDIT is an alcohol use screening tool developed in association with the World Health Organization (WHO), the results of which are linked to a decision process (Babor, Higgins-Biddle, Saunders, & Monteiro, 2001). AUDIT items cover amount and frequency of drinking, alcohol dependence, and problems caused by drinking.
- **Mood Disorders Questionnaire** (MDQ; Hirschfeld et al., 2000): Items on the MDQ correspond to the *DSM-IV* criteria for bipolar disorder.
- **National Initiative for Children's Health Care Quality's Vanderbilt ADHD Rating Scales** (Wolraich, Feurer, Hannah, Baumgaertel, & Pinnock, 1998): This ADHD assessment tool contains both parent and teacher rating scales. The items correspond to *DSM-IV* criteria for ADHD. The tool also contains screens for commonly co-occurring behavioral health conditions such as behavior disorders and depression/anxiety while also providing ADHD-related severity scores.

These questionnaires were selected not only because they are well known and have been shown to be valid and reliable but because they are relatively easy to use, are applicable to conditions frequently seen by mental health providers, and are in the public domain. Thus, you should have no trouble finding any of these instruments on the internet.

By utilizing outcome measures such as symptom severity questionnaires, you can document quality to MCOs. More and more MCOs are looking to incorporate outcome measurement into their management of providers. By taking the initiative to use outcome measures in treatment plans, you can increase your appeal to MCOs. Having data on progress in care can also be helpful when requesting additional sessions. Some questionnaires, like the PHQ-9 for depression, have the added benefit of including an item about suicidal ideation. By routinely giving this questionnaire, you can also document that you asked about and reviewed suicidal ideation, which is also very important to MCOs because of its risk to life and because it is a strong predictor of hospitalization (Pacificare Behavioral Health, 2001a). Similarly, incorporating a substance abuse screening tool like the AUDIT into your work ensures that you will be aware of your patient's alcohol use, which is also very important to MCOs who understand that alcohol and other drug abuse are associated with increased health problems and missed days of work (Schneider Institute for Health Policy, 2001).

Offering Treatment That Is in Demand

While high-quality treatment is always in demand, you can increase your appeal to an MCO and generate additional referrals by offering treatment and services that are in demand. The first step is to find out what types of services are most needed and which populations are most underserved. It is a good idea to review an MCO's list of providers, paying particular attention to their specialties and locations. Try to identify what specialties are in greatest demand and if possible (and appropriate) market yourself as a provider with a specialty in those areas and be sure to inform the MCO's provider relations department. The type of treatment in demand will vary greatly by MCO and geographic location. Generally speaking, however, mental health providers (particularly psychiatrists) who specialize in working with children are currently in high demand. Similarly, those with experience providing care to the elderly and to people with serious and persistent mental illness also appear to be in demand. In addition to specialty, pay close attention to geographical needs. If you notice a geographic area that is covered by few providers, consider trying to provide services in that area and let the MCO's provider relations department know about your ability to do so.

Summary Tips

- Know each of the NCQA HEDIS measures.
- Identify your patients meeting criteria for these measures as early as possible.
- Provide the quickest possible access to posthospitalized patients.
- Emphasize the importance of keeping appointments to your patients and document having done so.

- Emphasize the importance of proper medication adherence to your patients and document having done so.
- Collaborate with prescribing physicians or other treating providers.
- Inform provider relations when you are having difficulty contacting a patient or need help for the patient to achieve treatment adherence.
- Incorporate outcome-based measures such as symptom questionnaires into your treatment.
- Read all of the MCO's behavioral health clinical practice guidelines.
- Anticipate measures to be used to monitor those clinical practice guidelines.

CHAPTER TEN

Generating Business From Within the Managed Care System

In the previous chapter, techniques for generating referrals from the MCO through the demonstration of quality or providing treatment that is in demand were presented. This chapter also focuses on building your practice by generating increased referrals, this time by using the MCO's system proactively in order to generate referrals as opposed to waiting for the MCO to make referrals to you. Being a part of an MCO's network of providers presents opportunities to greatly expand your practice, yet many providers do not take advantage of this opportunity. The best opportunity for expansion within the MCO system lies with partnering with medical providers in primary (and multispecialty) care practices to provide behavioral health care. While this may seem like a simple proposition, doing it correctly in a way that is likely to generate significant referrals involves several key components: developing relationships with PCPs, communicating effectively with PCPs, and identifying other physicians for collaboration.

Developing Relationships With PCPs

Most mental health care, especially depression care, is now provided by PCPs as opposed to specialty care providers (Coyne et al., 2002; U.S. Department of Health and Human Services, 1993). Despite the high volume of mental health treatment being provided by PCPs, studies show that much of this care is at suboptimal or inadequate levels (Finley et al., 2003; U.S. Department of Health and Human

Services, 1993). Studies also show that most PCPs would welcome the opportunity to work collaboratively with mental health specialists to provide treatment for mental health conditions (Brazeau, Rovi, Yick, & Johnson, 2005; Kolbasovsky et al., 2005). When you take these findings together with the fact that as a provider for an MCO you are part of a team of mental health and medical providers working to provide care for its members, you begin to see the vast potential for partnering and collaborating with medical providers to provide mental health care. With most physicians scheduling four patients per hour and as many as 20–50% of patients presenting in primary care having a mental health issue (Collaborative Family Healthcare Coalition, 1998; Olfson et al., 1997; White, 1997), it is easy to see how partnering with a few physicians can generate a vast number of new referrals to your practice. The question then becomes how to make it happen. This section includes a series of steps designed to help you use the managed care system to develop collaborative relationships with physicians in order to quickly and effectively build your practice.

Step 1: Identify Physicians in Your Network to Target for Collaboration

The first thing you should do is get a copy of the list of providers for the MCO for which you are a mental health provider. Simply call the MCO and request that they mail you a copy if you do not already have one and it is not available online. Once you get the list, you will probably find that hundreds if not thousands of medical providers are listed. Clearly you cannot try to partner with all of these medical providers, so you will need to narrow your focus. The first step in narrowing your focus is to identify physicians practicing in your area. Obviously, a physician is more likely to refer a patient to you if you are close. Similarly, a referred patient is more likely to actually appear for an appointment if that appointment is located close to where he or she is used to getting medical services.

After narrowing the list to medical providers practicing close to you, you may find that there are still many providers on the list. So whom do you target to approach about initiating a collaborative relationship? You could send a letter to every provider informing him or her that you provide mental health services in the area, are on the same MCO panel, and are interested in receiving referrals. However, a low-intensity outreach like this by itself is not likely to have much of an impact on the number of new referrals you generate. You could also just randomly pick out a select number of providers to target for a more intense outreach, but luckily certain physician characteristics predict a greater likelihood of interest in collaborating with mental health providers.

Female physicians, younger physicians, and physicians residency-trained in family practice are more likely to be interested in collaborating with you as a mental health provider (Brazeau et al., 2005; Robinson, Geske, Prest, & Barnacle, 2004). Female physicians are reported to engage in more psychosocial counseling and question-asking than their male counterparts, suggesting that they may be better at identifying and referring patients for mental health conditions (Roter, Hall, & Aoki, 2002). Female PCPs are also more likely to suggest combination therapy (medication and psychotherapy as opposed to just medication) than their male counterparts (Robinson et al., 2004) making them particularly attractive potential collaborative partners for therapists. Younger and family practice-trained physicians may also be more comfortable collaborating with mental health specialists due to greater experience with these providers during their family medicine residency training (Brazeau et al., 2005). At least in one study, family practitioners were more likely to have more female patients than internal medicine physicians (Robinson et al., 2004). This may be important as female patients are probably more likely to accept a referral to mental health treatment than males. Keep in mind that these trends should not be taken to indicate that other types of physicians would not also welcome the opportunity to collaborate. These trends are simply offered to help you target medical providers with whom you may be most likely to generate the greatest number of referrals.

The next question becomes, how do you use these findings to help direct your search? Luckily, most of the information you need should be available from the MCO provider lists. These lists typically indicate the name location, and specialty of each physician. In some cases, you may also be able to find out the number of years they have been in practice (which can be used as a proxy for age). If the information is not available, you may consider placing a call to the physician's office directly and ask the support staff member these types of general questions about the physician and his or her practice. Once you have this information, it should not be difficult to identify several physicians practicing in a location near you that have a specialty in family practice, are female, or both. You may even be able to target younger clinicians if the information is available. While such physicians may generally speaking be quite receptive to collaboration with mental health providers, these should not be considered the only types of physicians who would be receptive. You should not hesitate to include other types of physicians in your list as well. Select other specialists to target based on the types of mental health conditions they are likely to come across most frequently and your comfort level in treating those conditions. A nonexhaustive list of physician specialties and the mental health conditions they are likely to come across follows:

- **Obstetricians and gynecologists (OB/GYN):** Approximately 10% of mothers experience postpartum depression (Epperson, 1999; Georgiopoulos et al., 1999). Recent years have also seen an increase in the number of women seeking help for depression, anxiety, and somatoform disorders (Cassidy, Boyle, & Lawrence, 2003). In addition, the American College of Obstetrics and Gynecology stated that the college must expand its vision beyond reproduction to embrace conditions disproportionately affecting the quality of life for women, such as depression (Cassidy et al., 2003).
- **Endocrinologists:** People with diabetes experience twice the rate of depression as people without diabetes (Lustman et al., 2000) and depression is associated with elevated risk of diabetes complications (Forrest, Becker, Kuller, Wolfson, & Orchard, 2000; Lustman, 1988; Lustman et al., 2000; Peyrot & Rubin, 1999; Zhang et al., 2005). Anger and stress are also common issues that may impact the course of a person's diabetes and the ability to self-manage the condition (Kolbasovsky, 2004; McCord & Brandeburg, 1995; Peyrot & Rubin, 1999; Snoek, 2002).
- **Internal Medicine Physicians:** Internal medicine doctors see a wide range of mental conditions presenting in their offices.
- **Cardiologists:** People with heart disease are more likely to suffer from depression than those without heart disease and people with depression are at higher risk for developing heart disease (Frassure-Smith, Lesperance, & Talajic, 1995). In addition, people who are depressed have a higher risk of death after a heart attack compared to those who are not depressed (Frasure-Smith, Lesperance, & Talajic, 1995).
- **Pediatricians:** ADHD is the most common mental health condition seen in children (Richters et al., 1995) and pediatricians are the health care providers families tend to turn to first for treatment, even though many pediatricians do not feel comfortable diagnosing or treating ADHD (Miller, Johnston, Klassen, Fine, & Papsdorf, 2005).

SPOTLIGHT ON

Doctors Seeking Collaboration

A psychologist brought his newborn daughter to her first appointment with her pediatrician. After the pediatrician completed her examination, she noticed that the patient's father had indicated a profession of "psychologist" on the initial paperwork. She then asked him if he saw children in his practice because the group of pediatricians was having great difficulty connecting children with mental health care. The psychologist had only been considering developing a part-time private practice at the time but saw a need that he could fill. He began a collaborative relationship with the group of pediatricians and started to see fee-for-service patients while working to get on the same managed care panels as the pediatricians. Within several months, he was able to join several MCOs and continued to receive many referrals from his daughter's pediatricians.

Step 2: Contacting Potential Physician Partners

Once you have generated your list, you will need to contact these physicians to inform them that you are in practice, are contracted with the same MCO they are, and are interested in receiving referrals. You will also want to communicate the benefits to the physician and his or her patients of building a collaborative relationship with you. Mental health providers often make the mistake of simply making one call to a physician, leaving one message or sending one letter, and then expect to start receiving referrals from that physician. Keep in mind that most physicians are very busy and are less likely to refer to someone with whom they are not personally familiar (McNeil, 2000). After all, would you refer your patients to a physician you did not know anything about? Developing a collaborative relationship that begins to generate referrals is not a one-time event. You will need to continuously work on this relationship (Kolbasovsky & Reich, 2005). A more appropriate opening strategy would be to call each physician that you have targeted and arrange to go to that physician's medical center to meet briefly in person at a time that is convenient for the physician, most likely during a lunch hour or at the end of the day. This may seem time consuming and inconvenient to you, and it is, but this sends an important message to the physician that you are willing to go the extra mile. It also gives the physician a chance to actually get to know you. In the long run, steps like this are key to generating referrals and building collaborative relationships.

Step 3: The In-Person Meeting

When meeting with a physician, be respectful of the physician's time and be brief yet friendly. Explain exactly how you can help with the diagnosis and treatment of mental health conditions that should be fairly common in the physician's practice. You should be familiar with exactly what types of conditions are most common in that physician's specialty. Try to generate a brief discussion about what mental health conditions the physician sees most frequently. You may also want to briefly discuss your approach to treating those conditions. If the physician is amenable, you can also discuss brief screenings that can be used in primary care to detect possible mental health conditions in need of referral. A brief, nonexhaustive list of possible screens for use in primary care follows:

- US Preventive Services Task Force's (2002) two-question screen:
  1. Over the past 2 weeks, have you felt down, depressed, or hopeless?
  2. Over the past 2 weeks, have you felt little interest or pleasure in doing things?
- Brief Diagnostic Screen for Panic Disorder in Primary Care: Autonomic Nervous System Questionnaire (Stein et al., 1999):
  1. In the past 6 months, did you ever have a spell or attack when all of a sudden you felt frightened, anxious, or very uneasy?
  2. In the past 6 months, did you ever have a spell or attack when for no reason your heart suddenly began to race, you felt faint, or you couldn't catch your breath?
- Primary Care PTSD Screen (Prins et al., 1999):
  In your life, have you ever had any experience that was so frightening, horrible, or upsetting that in the past month you . . .
  1. Have had nightmares about the event when you did not want to? (Yes/No)
  2. Tried hard not to think about it or went out of your way to avoid situations that reminded you of it? (Yes/No)
  3. Were constantly on guard, watchful, or easily startled? (Yes/No)
  4. Felt numb or detached from others, activities, or your surroundings? (Yes/No)
- CAGE screen (Ewing, 1984) for alcohol abuse:
  1. Have you ever felt you ought to *cut* down on your drinking?
  2. Have people *annoyed* you by criticizing your drinking?
  3. Have you ever felt *guilty* about your drinking?
  4. Have you ever had a drink first thing in the morning as an *eye*-opener?

After a brief discussion about mental health conditions and how you can help to treat them, be sure to mention what insurance you accept as that will be important information for patients. Explain also that you place a great emphasis on communicating information to the PCP and that you will (with the patient's consent) provide feedback to the physician on an ongoing basis, welcome information and questions from the referring physician, and make yourself available to that physician to collaborate on all patients referred. This is vital, as lack of feedback from mental health specialists is a common complaint of physicians (Gandhi et al., 2000; McNeil, 2000). Physicians feel a great sense of urgency when referring for mental health conditions, yet are frequently dissatisfied with the amount of communication they receive from mental health providers (Little et al., 1998). It is this commitment to communication and collaboration that will generate referrals to you in the future. As you end the meeting, you may also want to explain your treatment philosophy and ways in which you typically practice. Be sure to leave the physician with plenty of business cards or flyers that can be handed out to patients who need to set up an appointment. Make sure that you are brief, informative, and friendly. Keep in mind that you are selling yourself and your practice to the physician.

Step 4: The Thank-You

Shortly after your meeting, be sure to call and thank the physician for meeting with you. Not only is this polite, it serves to start building your relationship and it reminds the physician that you are available and eager to provide collaborative mental health care. You should also strongly consider sending a thank-you letter or e-mail as well. Keep in mind that in the beginning, before you start to receive referrals, you may need to come up with reasons for contacting the physician, just to remind him or her that you are available for referrals, and a thank-you for the meeting is a good way to maintain contact without appearing pushy.

Step 5: The Follow-up

Do not expect that you will suddenly start getting many referrals. The process of generating referrals is often slow at first. You should periodically call the physicians with whom you have initiated a relationship. Remind them of your desire to partner with them and your availability to take referrals. You may want to mention that you recently came across a good article related to something you spoke about in your meeting (e.g., screening for depression in primary care, or assessing suicide risk) that you thought they might be interested in reading. Then ask if you can send a copy. In your discussions with physicians, keep an ear out for any challenges or difficulties a physician voices related to mental health, then find ways of helping that physician. Even if your help in that situation does not directly generate any business for you, by helping the physician you are building a better relationship and you will be more likely to get referrals in the future as you are building trust and demonstrating competency with that physician.

Step 6: Handling the Referral and Maintaining Communication

When you receive a referral, be sure to provide the fastest possible access to an appointment, the highest possible quality of care, and the best possible customer service. You will be judged by how you handle early referrals. Make sure that you ask the referred patient to sign a consent form allowing for collaboration with the referring physician. Be sure to explain to the patient exactly why this is so important. After your initial consultation, be sure to send the referring physician written feedback and also call to provide verbal feedback and a thank-you for the referral. If you foresee any ways in which the behavioral health condition may impact the patient's medical condition or ability to self-manage that condition, be sure to discuss this with the physician. You can also ask the physician if he or she has made any medical recommendations to the patient that you should follow up on (e.g., lose weight, begin to exercise, schedule an MRI, improve adherence to medication), particularly because following medical recommendations can often have very positive effects on mental health conditions as well.

Throughout the treatment process, you should provide feedback to the referring physician both in writing and verbally. This allows for greater collaboration and reminds the physician that you are available to handle additional referrals. It is likely you will get a small number of referrals at first, but that is likely to increase rapidly once the physician has received positive feedback from patients about you (thus, you should do all you can to provide a positive experience to all patients) and you have developed more of a collaborative relationship with that physician (Kolbasovsky et al., 2005). Keep in mind that most physicians want feedback about their patients in an ongoing fashion. Be sure to develop a system whereby you will contact each referring physician to provide feedback and further develop your working relationship, not just upon consultation but throughout the treatment process. There are many opportune times to provide feedback to a PCP. For example, Magellan Behavioral Health (2004) recommends sending information to physicians in the following situations:

- Following the member's initial evaluation.
- At the time of any significant change in the member's status, such as a psychiatric hospitalization.

SPOTLIGHT ON

The Follow-up

A psychologist utilizing the steps outlined in this chapter met in person, over lunch with a group of physicians who worked together in the same medical center. One of the physicians, a young female with a specialty in family medicine, happened to mention that she had recently diagnosed several patients with acute stress disorder. During the conversation, it quickly became clear that this physician had an excellent relationship with her patients, took the time to actually get to know them, and had at least some interest in addressing mental health issues. It also turned out that she was using "acute stress disorder" to mean someone who was dealing with a current life stressor and not someone who had recently experienced a traumatic event and was experiencing symptoms associated with that trauma. The psychologist explained the difference in terms and later followed up by mailing the physician some additional information on trauma, anxiety, and adjustment disorders, including a few questions to help differentiate between the conditions. Very soon, the physician made quite a few referrals to the psychologist. The psychologist sent a great deal of feedback to the physician on the cases she referred and before long a mutually beneficial collaborative relationship developed, resulting a substantial increase in referrals to the psychologist's practice. The lesson here is to look for opportunities to provide physicians with information that is practical and helpful to them in working with their patients. Going above and beyond the call of duty for a provider who has the potential to make referrals to you can make a huge financial difference to your practice.

- Whenever psychiatric medications are initiated or treatment or diagnosis indicates medication.
- Following any significant changes in medication.

It is always important to provide information and collaborate with physicians sending you referrals. However, in some cases it may be of even greater importance. BHN (2005) lists several types of patients for whom communication with the PCP is particularly important:

- Patients with high utilization of general medical services or chronic medical conditions.
- Patients referred to a behavioral health provider by a PCP.
- Patients on psychotropic medication or narcotic pain medication.
- Patients with an eating disorder.
- Patients with chronic pain.

In addition to helping you to generate referrals, communication with PCPs is often a measure that MCOs use to rate mental health providers. Since MCOs may choose any subtype of members and then evaluate mental health providers as to their rate of communicating feedback to the PCP, your best approach is to send feedback initially and throughout treatment to your patients' PCPs, thus ensuring compliance with all MCOs.

Physician Communication

Collaboration with physicians can be achieved only through ongoing communication. MCOs understand that proper communication between mental health providers and medical providers is critical to providing high-quality continuous care. This is why almost all MCOs will strongly request that you send a communication form to a member's PCP following your first visit with that member. Almost all MCOs will even provide the communication form, typically including it as part of the provider's manual. These forms vary but typically include member background information, diagnosis, psychotropic medication, and treatment recommendations. Of course, you should get patient consent prior to sending information to the PCP.

Despite the importance of this communication to both mental health and medical treatment, and the vast potential of growing their practices through partnership with physicians, a substantial number of providers do not even bother to send a communication form to their patients' PCPs. In fact, Magellan (2004) reported that record reviews of high-volume providers showed that the rate of PCP communication (as evidenced by a single written communication form sent to a PCP) was only 45% in 2002 and that the rate rose to 63% in 2003 only after several interventions were implemented to improve communication. Magellan concluded that there is opportunity for greater improvement. Similarly, BHN (2005) reported that recent quality improvement activities helped to raise the rate of communication between prescribing mental health providers and PCPs from less than 50% in 2002 to 73% in 2004. The lesson here is that communication with PCPs is highly valued by MCOs and plays a critical part in building your practice, yet many providers still fail to take advantage of this opportunity.

The role of communication with medical providers should not be overlooked when it comes to growing your practice. A study of almost 1,000 referrals found referring physicians' satisfaction ratings were significantly increased when they received any type of specialist feedback (Forrest et al., 2000). Information these physicians seemed to appreciate most was suggestions for future care, follow-up arrangements, and plans for comanaging care. When possible, you should be sure to incorporate this information into your communication with referring medical providers. Another study involving telephone surveys found that 54% of the over 6,500 PCPs surveyed reported having problems arranging outpatient mental health referrals (Trude & Stoddard, 2003). This problem was particularly marked for pediatricians. This finding should signal to you that mental health providers are needed by medical providers and that mental health providers who can ease the process of connecting medical patients to mental health care should generate a great many referrals.

To summarize, medical practitioners see a very high volume of patients with mental health conditions (White, 1997). Yet for many of these patients the behavioral health condition goes undetected or undertreated. Collaborative treatment between medical and behavioral health providers has been shown to lead to improved outcomes (Katon, Von Korff, & Lin, 1995) and many physicians would be interested in forming collaborative relationships with mental health providers if given the opportunity (Brazeau et al., 2005). Therefore, partnering with medical providers provides you with a wealth of opportunity to generate new referrals to build your practice and generate greater revenue.

Identifying Other Physicians for Collaboration

Other physicians who are often overlooked are the physicians providing care to patients you are already treating. These physicians may or may not be on the same MCO panels as you, which could limit their ability to make referrals, but they should not be overlooked. Since you are already treating their patients, you simply need to take the appropriate steps to identify them, obtain your patients' consent, and contact the physicians directly. A patient's PCP and the contact information can often be found on the patient's MCO identification card, by contacting the MCO's provider relations department, or by looking the information up on the MCO's Web site (if that option is available). Upon contacting the PCP, you can introduce yourself and then begin to provide relevant feedback. As you build a collaborative relationship with these physicians, you should not have a difficult time generating referrals in the future.

In addition to forging collaborative relationships with physicians treating your patients, think of any physicians you may already know personally that could be a source of referral to you. A good place to start is with physicians that provide medical care to you and your family. Chances are you (or members of your family) have seen the same doctor for a number of years and have a good relationship with that doctor. You may want to consider talking with your PCP, OB/GYN, other specialist, or your child's pediatrician about becoming a mental health resource for that physician. The relationship and trust you and your family have built with that physician may go a long way in generating referrals and growing your practice.

SPOTLIGHT ON

Identifying Other Physicians for Collaboration

A psychologist working full-time at a state hospital became pregnant and made the decision to leave her position at the hospital. She did not want to stop working completely but needed a job where she could work flexible hours around her husband's schedule once her baby was born. She made the decision to start a private practice even though she had no referral sources. During one of her routine OB/GYN appointments, she happened to mention to her doctor her plans and her concern for the future. Her doctor mentioned that she was frequently confronted with mental health issues, particularly depression, and lacked resources. Several months later, the psychologist gave birth to a healthy baby girl. A few months after that, the psychologist started her part-time private practice and received several referrals from her OB/GYN.

Summary Tips

- Partner with your MCO's medical providers to generate referrals.
- Use recent findings to target medical providers.

- Target only a limited number of physicians but invest significant time and energy in building your relationship with those physicians.
- Be sensitive to the time demands of physicians.
- Be alert for any ways you can provide assistance to a physician on a behavioral health issue even before you are referred any patients.
- Consider giving screening tools to physicians to help them identify behavioral health conditions in need of treatment.
- Emphasize physician communication for all of your patients.
- Provide ongoing feedback to and collaboration with PCPs.
- Explain the importance of collaboration to your patients.
- Form collaborative relationships with physicians treating your current patients.

CHAPTER ELEVEN

Practice Opportunities: Future Directions of Managed Care

Predicting the future is always an arduous task, particularly when it comes to trying to stay ahead of the very fast-paced and ever-changing world of managed health care in the United States. Despite the inherent difficulties, this chapter discusses the likely future directions of managed care and what those directions will mean to mental health providers. Given the current state of managed care and the challenges that lie ahead, there will likely be many changes to the managed care system in the near future. Several of these changes should directly affect mental health providers, including continued and increased consolidation of managed care companies, increased reintegration of mental health into MCOs, expansion of disease management, greater mental health integration with primary care medical providers, increased opportunities for providers in behavioral medicine, increased role of technology in private practice, increased opportunities to practice outside of the traditional office, increased expectation in the use of outcome measures, and an expanded focus on reducing disparities in health care.

Consolidation of Managed Care Companies

Recent years have witnessed a consolidation of managed care companies, with fewer and fewer companies covering more and more members. Many experts expect that this trend will continue as large MCOs continue to acquire smaller ones (AIS Market Data, 2004). This trend is likely to result in relatively few managed care companies managing health care for most Americans. Just how few MCOs will ultimately remain is of course unknown. However, with fewer MCOs covering a greater and greater percentage of the population, there will be increased pressure on mental health providers interested in working with managed care to join the network of one or more of these large MCOs. Failing to become a provider for these large MCOs could make it difficult to generate business for your practice. For example, if you are on the panel of a smaller MCO in your area and a larger MCO acquires that MCO as well as others, you may no longer be able to see your patients unless you become credentialed by the larger MCO. Similarly, if a large MCO suddenly covers 80% of the people with health care coverage in your area and you are not in that network, generating business may become quite difficult. Luckily, having read this book, you are well prepared not only to join managed care networks but to thrive in the managed care environment.

With the continued consolidation of health plans, MCOs are likely to gain even greater power when negotiating with providers. It is not surprising that many providers may feel a sense of diminished power and a fear of being excluded from MCO networks if they fail to conform to the company's norms and expectations (Mechanic, 1999). While increased pressure to conform to the demands of MCOs will not likely be viewed as something positive by mental health providers, one potentially positive aspect of this consolidation may be greater uniformity in the industry. For example, instead of having to complete several different forms for the several different MCOs you may currently be working with, in the future you may only need to work with one or two MCOs who most likely will have similar forms that have become standard in the industry. The simplification of this process may then allow mental health providers to put more of their time and energies into working billable hours and less into paperwork.

Reintegration of Mental Health Into MCOs

While most mental health care coverage is now managed by carve-out organizations, the current trend toward bringing mental health management back in-house is likely to continue (Duck, 2005). Bringing mental health in-house has the potential for improving the integration of mental health and medical services, which may be particularly important as the costs of psychiatric medication, a component of care that is often not managed by carve-outs, represent a significant portion of managed care pharmacy expenditures (Duckworth & Hanson, 2002; Harrington et al., 2000). The reintegration of mental health should make it easier for mental health providers to collaborate with medical providers, thus potentially improving the overall quality of care to the MCO's members. As this trend continues, providers should be aware that greater importance is being placed on collaboration with medical providers and should have processes in place to make sure they are engaging in collaboration with PCPs on a routine basis throughout treatment. The rate at which this reintegration will occur remains to be seen and will of course be influenced greatly by the ability of MCOs to demonstrate greater costeffectiveness and greater overall quality of care while managing mental health benefits in-house.

Expansion of Disease Management

Along with a trend toward bringing the management of mental health benefits inhouse has come the growth and expansion of disease management. According to the Disease Management Association of America (2006), disease management is defined as a system of coordinated health care interventions and communications for populations with conditions in which patient self-care efforts are significant. Disease management supports the physician or specialist provider-patient relationship and plan of care, emphasizes prevention of exacerbations and complications utilizing evidence-based practice guidelines and patient empowerment strategies, and evaluates outcomes on an ongoing basis to improve overall health (Disease Management Association of America, 2006). As you can see from the definition, disease management places great emphasis on the proper management of a condition. Disease management often involves the use of a disease manager who may also be referred to as a coach or a case manager. Using a disease management approach, an MCO or a separate company contracted to provide disease management services for a specific condition will identify the MCO's members with that condition and provide appropriate services. Often these services may involve screening for mental health conditions and referrals to mental health providers as needed, telephonic and mailed reminders of appointments to members, facilitation collaboration between providers, and pharmacy management. Pharmacy management may involve such interventions as reminder calls when refills are due, monitoring medication adherence, and monitoring provider prescription practices.

In response to this growing trend toward the reintegration of mental health, traditional mental health carve-out companies will likely move toward providing disease management as opposed to strictly managing mental health benefits. For example, at a conference, the chief clinical officer for Magellan Health Services, a company that is no longer providing carve-out mental health management for Aetna, discussed the need for greater disease and pharmacy management within managed care (Kotin, 2006). Similarly, in 2005, APS Healthcare, known for its management of mental health, was awarded the Disease Management Association of America's Recognizing Excellence Award for Best Government Disease Management Program (DM World e-Report, 2006). As a mental health provider in an era witnessing the growth of disease management, you should be prepared to receive referrals from disease managers and should be prepared to collaborate with them. Since disease management staff members can be a potentially lucrative source of referrals, mental health providers looking to build their practices should work on developing positive working relationships with disease managers.

Integration of Mental Health and Primary Care

As studies continue to show that more and more people are receiving mental health care, particularly for depression and anxiety disorder, in primary care rather than specialty mental health care settings, and that the mental health treatment provided in primary care is frequently suboptimal, greater integration of primary care and mental health specialists is likely to continue (Coyne et al., 2002; Finley et al., 2004; U.S. Department of Health and Human Services, 1993). You should be aware that in the future you as a mental health provider will likely see an even greater emphasis on demonstrating that you are actively collaborating with your patient's PCP. As outside evaluative agencies continue to require monitoring of this collaboration and as MCOs realize the need to improve the quality of mental health care delivered, more and more scrutiny will be placed on collaboration. Therefore, you should make sure that you already have an efficient system in place for sending and documenting written and verbal information to the PCPs of your patients.

In addition to the increasing importance of documenting collaboration, the continued integration of primary care and mental health should bring new opportunities for mental health providers. In fact, several studies that collocated mental health specialists into primary care medical facilities to work collaboratively with physicians to deliver mental health care have documented the abilities of such arrangements to deliver high-quality care (Beck, 2001; Coyne et al., 2002; Finley et al., 2003; Gill & Dansky, 2003; Kanapaux, 2004; Katon, Russo, & Von Korff, 2002; Katon, Von Korff, & Lin, 1997; Katon et al., 1995; Kolbasovsky et al., 2005). As new roles for mental health providers open up in primary care, those best suited to fill the positions will have a demonstrated history of collaborating and developing relationships with medical providers. Therefore, you should not wait to begin getting to know (with consent) the PCPs of your patients, particularly any physicians who may also be prescribing psychiatric medication to your patients.

Opportunities in Behavioral Medicine

As mental health providers are further integrated and collocated into primary care medical centers, increased opportunities for providers should develop in the arena of behavioral medicine. Within the context of managed care, behavioral medicine involves the use of psychological or behavioral interventions to impact on medical as well as psychological outcomes. Because many chronic medical conditions are either caused by or mediated by behaviors such as poor eating habits, sedentary lifestyles, smoking, and poor medication management, mental health providers with an expertise in behavior change are in an ideal position to help individuals with chronic medical conditions make these needed behavior and lifestyle changes. Already mental health providers have demonstrated the ability to improve medical outcomes for individuals with diabetes and cardiovascular diseases. For example, adult MCO members with diabetes completing a structured group-based program led by mental health providers demonstrated statistically significant reductions in HbA1c level (a measure of average glucose level over a 3-month period) after completion of the program (Kolbasovsky, 2005). Similarly, a study of people in cardiac rehabilitation found that psychological interventions targeting self-regulatory skills can enable postrehabilitation patients to reduce behavioral risk factors and facilitate intended lifestyle changes (Sciehotta et al., 2005).

As studies continue to demonstrate improved medical outcomes associated with behavioral interventions delivered by mental health providers, more and more MCOs will look to take advantage of this opportunity. As they do, more reimbursement opportunities for mental health providers should be created. The opportunities will likely be most available to providers already integrated into medical settings, as they will have easier access to referrals and will have an easier time developing collaborative relationships with medical providers. While the development of opportunities in behavioral medicine within the managed care environment may take some time, this emerging field holds exciting opportunities for mental health providers and brings health care one step closer to greater appreciation of the mind-body connection.

Practice Opportunities Outside of the Traditional Office

In addition to new opportunities for mental health providers in medical settings, there will likely be new practice opportunities for providers outside of the traditional office. As you are aware, NCQA and other evaluative agencies use measures that often involve the percentage of members seen within a given time frame. For example, MCOs are often judged on the percentage of members hospitalized for a psychiatric condition that are seen for an outpatient follow-up appointment within 7 days of discharge. One large barrier to success on this type of measure is that some members are unable to attend an appointment in a provider's office because of physical limitations that prevent them from traveling or even leaving home, or financial limitations that prevent them from owning a car or being able to pay for public transportation. These problems are likely even more pronounced in rural areas where travel options are more limited and providers are more distant. These physical and financial limitations are probably most likely to affect elderly members and members from low socioeconomic backgrounds, two groups that are traditionally underserved when it comes to mental health care. To overcome these barriers, some MCOs are beginning to look for mental health providers who are willing to meet with members in the members' homes instead of the traditional office setting.

In the near future, more MCOs are likely to offer at least some opportunity for providers to be reimbursed for in-home visits. While this may create unique challenges for delivering care, it should improve access to care for people in need and at risk for falling through the cracks while also reducing provider costs associated with renting office space. If providing care to members outside of the traditional office setting sounds appealing to you, you should contact your MCO's provider relations department today and let them know that you are interested in doing home-based visits and that you want to know if you can be approved to do so. Even MCOs that have not yet set up a system for this may be interested in having a provider willing to do home visits. When speaking with an MCO's representative about doing home visits, you may be most likely to have success if you can emphasize the potential for your home visits to improve the MCO's HEDIS measures (assuming the MCO is accredited by NCQA or will be pursuing accreditation in the near future). You may even want to inform the MCO that you would be interested in contacting and trying to visit any member in your area who was not seen within 7 days of discharge from a psychiatric hospitalization if the MCO will provide you with the names and numbers of these members. You can also emphasize how your home visits have the potential to reduce health care disparities by improving access to the underserved and may also improve the MCO's performance on other quality indicators (if you are aware of other quality indicators that may be impacted).

The Role of Technology in Private Practice

Regardless of where tomorrow's mental health providers deliver care, technology is likely to play an important role. MCOs are allowing mental health providers to conduct more and more business via computer. Many MCOs now allow providers to submit and monitor claims electronically and to check member eligibility on a secure Web site. Because the use of this technology is more cost efficient to the MCO, more confidential, and has the potential to speed up the reimbursement process for providers, the use of computers and the internet will likely only become more and more commonplace in the near future.

As public attention continues to be focused on avoidable mistakes in health care, a greater proliferation of electronic medical records seems likely. Electronic medical records overcome the common problem of illegible records. They also reduce costs associated with creating and storing paper-based medical records. In facilities, electronic medical records also have the benefit of providing easier access to reports of medical care delivered by a variety of providers, allowing for greater integration between providers and an overall improved quality of care.

Outside of a facility setting, an electronic medical record has many other benefits for the private practitioner. Electronic records can be created to flag cases that meet criteria for certain quality measures such as the NCQA HEDIS measures. These flags can then help providers to track these cases better. Electronic records can also be used to track scores on outcome measures over time, creating graphs depicting each patient's improvement throughout the course of treatment. With so many potential benefits, you may be asking why electronic medical records are not more commonplace today. The main reason is probably the barrier of expense. Switching to an electronic system usually involves a large up-front cost for facilities, and the current cost may be prohibitive for many solo private practices. However, if the cost associated with owning an electronic system decreases in the future or new legislation requiring such system is enacted, electronic medical records will become more commonplace for mental health providers working with managed care.

The Role of Outcome Measures

Currently, many process-of-care measures are used by MCOs to monitor the quality of mental health care delivered by providers. The incorporation of specific outcome-of-care measures is less common. However, certain MCOs such as Pacificare and United Behavioral Health are beginning to demonstrate the ability to monitor treatment outcomes through the use of patient-completed questionnaires that are repeated throughout treatment. The usefulness of this information to monitor and help drive toward improved outcomes is such that more MCOs are likely to incorporate outcome measurement in the future. As this becomes more widespread, outpatient mental health providers will be asked to have their patients complete questionnaires that assess either general functioning or condition-specific symptoms. Once completed, the results would be sent to the MCO and managed in a database.

Probably the greatest obstacle to the incorporation of this kind of outcome measurement for MCOs is the time and expense involved in getting providers and patients to comply and having staff available to collect and manage all of the data. As electronic medical records and electronic submission of claims and other information become more widespread, MCOs may have an easier time requiring outcome measurement from providers, as providers would be able to electronically submit results to an MCO database. There is no telling how quickly most MCOs will adopt systems for outcome measurement. However, mental health providers that become comfortable with the use of outcome measurement now will be prepared to meet the challenge to monitor outcomes in the future managed care environment.

Reducing Disparities in Health Care

With the increased role of outside evaluative agencies in managed care, greater attention is being paid to identifying and reducing disparities in health care. Ethnic, gender, and age disparities in the quality of mental health care have been noted. Some notable findings are that African Americans, Hispanics, and Asian Indians with mental illnesses are less likely to use psychiatric drugs than whites with mental illnesses (Han & Liu, 2005). African Americans may also be less likely than whites to receive second-generation antipsychotics (Mallinger, Fischer, Brown, & Lamberti, 2006), and girls have been found less likely than boys to obtain needed treatment for externalizing behavior disorders, while middle children are less likely to obtain treatment for any mental health problem than are older, younger, or only children (Zimmerman, 2005).

It should also be noted that disparities in health care are by no means limited to mental health care. Studies have also found disparities in the quality of medical care provided. For example, one study found that African Americans as compared to whites had lower odds of receiving a Pap test, rectal exam, smoking cessation counseling, and mental health advice during primary care office visits (Franks, Fiscella, & Meldrum, 2005). One group that may be particularly vulnerable to disparities in medical treatment is people with mental health conditions. This was highlighted in a study finding that failure to meet diabetes performance measures was more common in patients with mental health conditions (Frayne et al., 2005). This study found that people with mental health conditions, particularly those with psychotic disorders, mania, substance use, and personality disorders were at higher risk for having no HbA1c testing, no low-density lipoprotein cholesterol testing, no eye examination, poor glycemic control, and poor lipid control.

While only a very small segment of the health disparities research can be presented here, it is clear that there is work to be done to ensure that all people have equal access to quality health care. MCOs with their vast databases of health information and ability to help connect people with needed care have the potential to help reduce disparities. How well they are able to do this in the future remains to be seen. Mental health providers looking to excel in the managed care environment of today and tomorrow should aim to develop culturally sensitive practices while remaining aware of health disparities and working to reduce them.

Mental health providers should also be aware that people with mental health conditions may be at risk for receiving suboptimal medical care. Thus, part of your mental health treatment can involve discussions about medical care. Particularly for people with chronic medical conditions such as diabetes and hypertension, mental health providers can help patients learn techniques for making lasting behavioral and lifestyle changes such as increasing activity and improving eating habits. Mental health providers may also need to teach patients assertiveness skills in order to promote confidence in advocating for needed services. Similarly, mental health providers can help patients identify barriers to proper self-care while teaching problem-solving skills to help overcome them. In short, mental health providers working in managed care have vast opportunities to help reduce health care disparities faced by their patients. Of course, properly addressing medical concerns will typically involve the need to communicate with your patient's PCP. This, as you have read, is something that MCOs have been working very hard at improving over the last few years and is expected by most evaluative agencies.

Summary Tips

This final chapter has attempted to predict the future of managed care as it relates to mental health providers based on the current context. While there can be no way of knowing exactly what the future holds, you can prepare yourself for success by:

- Paying attention to the consolidation of MCOs in your geographic area and being prepared to join the network of any MCO that through acquisition or merger may soon dominate the health coverage in your area.
- Getting into the habit of routinely collaborating with PCPs and other medical providers of your patients.
- Learning to work with MCO disease management departments to help members to receive a higher quality of overall health care.
- Seeking opportunities to work directly in the primary medical care setting.
- Developing mental health–based strategies for improving not only mental health outcomes but medical outcomes as well.
- Becoming familiar with the use of a computer and using all computer-based options available to you from the MCO, and when possible using electronic medical records.
- Exploring opportunities to deliver needed services outside of the traditional office environment, especially for members who may not be able to travel to your office.
- Incorporating the use of outcome measures into your clinical work even if it is not required to by your MCO.
- Looking for opportunities to help members at risk for suboptimal mental health or medical care get the services that they need.

Conclusion

Keep in mind that no matter how well prepared for the future you are, there will also be challenges associated with working with managed care such as the commonly cited paperwork, oversight, and delays in reimbursement. These challenges will lead some providers to leave managed care, preferring to limit their practices to self-pay patients. With the growth of managed care coverage and the consolidation of health care companies, in the future there is likely to be even greater pressure on providers to join the networks of large MCOs in order to maintain a healthy private practice.

By reading this book, you are now in a great position to join the networks of both large and small MCOs. With the strategies provided, you are now armed with an understanding of why MCOs do what they do, what they are looking for from providers, and what they must demonstrate to outside evaluative agencies. With this information, you can speak in a language that will be heard by most MCOs. In addition to joining an MCO's network of credentialed providers, you now know how to get your services approved and how to get reimbursed in the timeliest manner possible. The strategies outlined in this book will also help you to reduce your liability and to have successful outcomes on MCO-sponsored chart audits. While managed care presents many challenges to clinicians, the well-informed provider is well positioned to develop a clinically and financially rewarding relationship with managed care organizations.

References

Abille v. United States, 482 F. Supp. 703 (N.D. Cal. 1980).

Adler, L., & Cohen, J. (2004). Diagnosis and evaluation of adults with attention deficit/hyperactivity disorder. *Psychiatric Clinics of North America, 27*(2), 187–201.

Affinity Health Plan. (2004). *Provider newsletter.* Retrieved November 16, 2005, from http://www.affinityplan.org/pnewslett.asp.

AFSCME. (2003). Integrating primary care and behavioral health: The next frontier. Retrieved from www.afscme.org/pol-log/mcmh03.htm.

AIS Market Data. (2004). Retrieved December 12, 2005, from http://www.aishealth.com/MarketData/MCEnrollment/MCEnrol_mc01.html.

Akechi, T., Okuyama, T., Sugawara, Y., Shima, Y., Furukawa, T., & Uchitomi, Y. (2006). Screening for depression in terminally ill cancer patients in Japan. *Journal of Pain Symptom Management, 31*(1), 5–12.

American Academy of Pediatrics. (2000). Clinical practice guideline: Diagnosis and evaluation of the child with attention deficit/hyperactivity disorder. *Pediatrics, 105*(5), 1158–1170.

American Educational Research Association, American Psychological Association, National Council on Measurement in Education. (1990). *Standards for educational and psychological testing.* Washington, DC: Author.

American Psychiatric Association. (1994). *Diagnostic and statistical manual of mental disorders* (4th ed.). Washington, DC: Author.

American Psychiatric Association. (2002a). *Documentation of psychotherapy by psychiatrists.* APA document reference no. 200202. Washington, DC: Author.

American Psychiatric Association. (2002b). *Minimum necessary guidelines for third-party payers for psychiatric treatment.* APA document reference no. 200211. Washington, DC: Author.

American Psychiatric Association (2002c). Practice guidelines for the treatment of patients with major depressive disorders (2nd ed.). *Journal of Lifelong Learning in Psychiatry, 3*(1), 34–42.

Appleby, C. (1997). Meet John Doe: When patients show up ahead of paperwork, aggravation and unpaid bills usually follow. *Hospital Health Network, 71*(6), 66–70.

APS Healthcare. (2003). *Provider manual.* Retrieved August 2, 2005, from http://www.apshealthcare.com/providers/bhp/aps_providermanual2004.pdf.

APS Healthcare. (2004). *The source: Provider newsletter.* Retrieved November 16, 2005, from http://www.apshealthcare.com/infoproviders/behav_health_prov.htm

Arkansas Senior Medicare/Medicaid Patrol Training Materials. (2005). Mental health fraud and abuse. Retrieved December 15, 2005, from http://www.arkansas .gov/dhhs/aging/11-MentalHealthFraudAndAbuse.pdf.

Babor, T., Higgins-Biddle, J., Saunders, J., & Monteiro, M. (2001). *Alcohol use disorders identification test. World Health Organization* (2nd ed.). Retrieved January 16, 2006, from http://whqlibdoc.who.int/hq/2001/WHO_MSD_MSB_01. 6a.pdf.

Batten, H., Prottas, J., & Horgan, C. (1992). *Drug service research survey, final report: phase II.* Submitted by the Bigel Institute for Health Policy, Brandeis University, to the National Institute on Drug Abuse, Waltham, MA.

Beaudin, C. (2005, October). *Delivering beyond the essentials: Innovations in managed behavioral healthcare.* Paper presented at the Integrating Behavioral Healthcare Management conference, Chicago, IL.

Beaudin, C., Vigil, V., & Weber, S. (2004). Suicide risk assessment in an MCO. *Managed Care Interface, 17*(5), 39–44.

Beck, A. (July/August, 2001). Collaborative behavioral health in primary care. *Group Practice Journal,* 22–26.

BHN. (2005). *Provider manual.* Retrieved September 1, 2005, from www. bhn.com.

Boersma, K., & Linton, S. (2006). Psychological processes underlying the development of a chronic pain problem. *Clinical Journal of Pain, 22*(2), 160–166.

Bornstein, R. (2001). Clinical utility of the Rorschach inkblot method: Reframing the debate. *Journal of Personality Assessment, 77*(1), 39–47.

Boydell, K., Malcolmson, S., & Sikerbol, K. (1991). Early rehospitalization. *Canadian Journal of Psychiatry, 36*(10), 723–725.

Brazeau, C., Rovi, S., Yick, C., & Johnson, M. (2005). Collaboration between mental health professionals and family physicians: A survey of New Jersey family physicians. *Primary Care Companion Journal of Clinical Psychiatry, 7,* 12–14.

Brown, G., Jones, E., Betts, E., & Wu, J. (2003). Improving suicide risk assessment in a managed health care environment. *Crisis: The Journal of Crisis Intervention and Suicide Prevention, 24*(2), 49–55.

Brytan, H., & Davis, O. (1997). Managing behavioral health risks: Claims analysis and risk management considerations. *Vantage Point, 2*(2), 2–5.

Buchanan, A. (1997). The investigation of acting on delusions as a tool for risk assessment in the mentally disordered. *British Journal of Psychiatry, 170*(32), 12–16.

Bull, S., Hu, X., & Hunkeler, E. (2002). Discontinuation of use and switching of antidepressants: Influence of patient-physician communication. *Journal of the American Medical Association, 288*(11), 1403–1409.

Cassidy, J., Boyle, V., & Lawrence, H. (2003). Behavioral healthcare integration in obstetrics and gynecology. *Medscape General Mededicine, 5*(2), 41.

Center for Mental Health Services. (2005). *Principles for systems of managed care.* Retrieved December 19, 2005, from http://www.mentalhealth.samhsa.gov/publications/allpubs/MC96-61/default.asp.

Cigna Behavioral Health. (2002) *Cigna provider connection.* Retrieved November 16, 2005, from http://64.233.161.104/search?q=cache:DBo8-vkFJ2gJ:apps.cigna behavioral.com/web/basicsite/provider/newsAndLearning/newsletter/newsletter 2002Quarter1.pdf+provider+newsletter+behavioral+health&hl=en.

Cigna Behavioral Health. (2005). *Provider manual.* Retrieved November 25, 2005, from http://www.cigna.com/health/provider/medical/procedural/claim_pro cessing/index.html.

Claasen, C., Hughes, C., Gilfillan, S., McIntire, D., Roose, A., Lumpkin, M., et al. (2000). Toward a redefinition of psychiatric emergency. *Health Service Research, 35*(3), 735–754.

Cohen, J. (2003). Managed care and the evolving role of the clinical social worker in mental health. *Social Work, 48*(1), 34–43.

Collaborative Family Healthcare Coalition. (1998). *Mental Illness and the Family.* Retrieved July 15, 2005, from www.nmha.org/infoctr/factsheets/15.cfm.

Columbia University Medical Center. (2005). *HIPAA policies: Confidentiality of psychotherapy and personal notes.* Retrieved February 1, 2006, from http://www.cumc.columbia.edu/hipaa/policies/psychotherapy.html.

Community Behavioral HealthCare Network of Pennsylvania. (2004). *Provider manual.* Retrieved November 25, 2005, from http://www.cbhnp.org/oldwebsite/providers/2004_Provider_Manual.pdf.

Compton, S., Cuffel, B., Burns, B., & Goldman, W. (2000). Datapoints: Effects of changing from five to ten preauthorized outpatient sessions. *Psychiatric Services, 51,* 1223.

Conti, D., & Burton, W. (1994). Economic impact of depression in a workplace. *Journal of Environmental Medicine, 36,* 983–988.

Conwell, Y., & Duberstein, P. (2001). Suicide in elders. *Annals of the New York Academy of Science, 932,* 132–147.

Coyne, J. C., Thompson, R., Klinkman, M., & Nease, D. (2002). Emotional disorders in primary care. *Journal of Consulting and Clinical Psychology, 70*(3), 789–809.

Cuffel, B., Held, M., & Goldman, W. (2002). Predictive models and the effectiveness of strategies for improving outpatient follow-up under managed care. *Psychiatric Services,* 53, 1438–1443.

deGroot, M., Anderson, R., Freedland, K., Clouse, R., & Lustman, P. (2001). Association of depression and diabetes complications: A meta analysis. *Psychosomatic Medicine, 63*(4), 619–630.

Dhossche, D., & Ghani, S. (1998). A study on recidivism in the psychiatric emergency room. *Annals of Clinical Psychiatry, 10*(2), 59–67.

Disease Management Association of America. (2006). *Definition of disease management.* Retrieved January 23, 2006, from http://www.dmaa.org/definition.html.

DM World e-Report. (2006, January 18). APS Healthcare grows health management business. *International Disease Management Alliance e-Newsletter.*

Duck, P. (2005). *Behavioral healthcare: Past, present, and future. Medical Records Institute.* Retrieved January 3, 2006, from www.medrecinst.com/proceedings/c0000357.pdf.

Duckworth, K., & Hanson, A. (2002). Managed care: Using a clinical and evidence-based strategy to ensure access to psychiatric medications. *Psychiatric Services, 53,* 1231–1232.

Empana, P., Jouven, X., Lemaitre, R., Sotoodehnia, N., Rea, T., Raghunathan, T., Simon, G., et al. (2006). Clinical depression and risk of out-of-hospital cardiac arrest. *Archives of Internal Medicine, 166*(2), 195–200.

Epperson, C. (1999). Postpartum major depression: Detection and treatment. *American Family Physician, 59*(8), 2247–2254.

Ewing, J. A. (1984). Detecting alcoholism. The CAGE questionnaire. *Journal of the American Medical Association, 252,* 1905–1907.

Excellus Blue Cross Blue Shield Behavioral Health Policy. (2005). *Precertification process.* Retrieved November 1, 2005, from https://www.excellusbcbs.com/providers/patient_care/behavioral_health.shtml.

Feldman J., & Finguerra, L. (2001). Managed crisis care for suicidal patients. In J. Ellison (Ed.), *Treatment of suicidal patients in managed care* (pp. 15–38). Washington, DC: American Psychiatric Press.

Felthous, A. (1999). The clinician's duty to protect third parties. *Psychiatric Clinics of North America, 22*(1), 49–60.

Fendrick, A., & Chernew, M. (2006). Value-based insurance design: A "clinically sensitive" approach to preserve quality of care and contain costs. *American Journal of Managed Care, 12*(1), 18–20.

Finley, P., Rens, H., Pont, J., Gess, S., Louie, C., Bull, S., et al. (2003). Impact of a collaborative care model on depression in a primary care setting: A randomized control trial. *Pharmacotherapy, 23*(9), 1175–1185.

Forrest, C., Glade, G., Baker, A., Bocian, A., von Schrader, S., & Starfield, B. (2000). Coordination of specialty referrals and physician satisfaction with referral care. *Archives of Pediatric Adolescent Medicine, 154*(5), 499–506.

Forrest, K., Becker, D., Kuller, L., Wolfson, S., & Orchard, T. (2000). Are predictors of coronary heart disease and lower-extremity arterial disease in type 1 diabetes the same? A prospective study. *Atherosclerosis, 148*, 159–169.

Franks, P., Fiscella, K., & Meldrum, S. (2005). Racial disparities in the context of primary care office visits. *Journal of General Internal Medicine, 20*(7), 599–603.

Frasure-Smith, N., Lesperance, F., & Talajic, M. (1995). Depression and 18-month prognosis after myocardial infarction. *Circulation,* 91(4), 999–1005.

Frayne, S., Halanych, J., Miller, D., Wang, F., Lin, H., Pogach, L., et al. (2005). Disparities in diabetes care: Impact of mental illness. *Archives of Internal Medicine, 165*(22), 2631–2638.

Gabel, J., Claxton, G., Pickering, E., Whitmore, H., Dhont, K., Hawkins, S., et al. (2003). Health benefits in 2003: Premiums reach 13 year high as employers adopt new forms of cost sharing. *Health Affairs, 22*(5), 117–126.

Gandhi, T., Sittig, D., Franklin, M., Sussman, A., Fairchild, D., & Bates, D. (2000). Communication breakdown in the outpatient referral process. *Journal of General Internal Medicine, 15*(9), 626–631.

Garb, H. (2002). Practicing psychological assessment. *American Psychologist, 57*(11), 990–991.

Garb, H. (2003). Incremental validity and the assessment of psychopathology in adults. *American Psychologist, 15*(4), 508–520.

Garb, H., Wood, J., & Nezworski, M. (2001). Toward a resolution of the Rorschach controversy. *Psychological Assessment, 13*(4), 433–448.

Garfield, S. (2000). The Rorschach test in clinical diagnosis. *Journal of Clinical Psychology, 56*(3), 387–434.

Georgia Department of Community Health. (2005). *Fraud and abuse.* Retrieved November 20, 2006, from http://dch.georgia.gov/00/channel_title/0,2094,314467 11_39681242,00.html.

Georgiopoulos, A., Bryan, T., Yawn, B., Houston, M., Rummans, T., & Therneau, T. (1999). Population based screening for postpartum depression. *Obstetrics and Gynecology, 93*(5), 653–637.

Gill, J. M., & Dansky, B. S. (2003). Use of an electronic medical record to facilitate screening for depression in primary care. *Primary Care Companion Journal of Clinical Psychiatry, 5*(3), 125–128.

Goldman, W., McCullouch, M., & Cuffel, B. (2003). A four-year study of enhancing outpatient psychotherapy in managed care. *Psychiatric Services, 54,* 41–49.

Groth-Marnat, G. (1999). Financial efficacy of clinical assessment: Rational guidelines and issues for further research. *Journal of Clinical Psychology, 55*(7), 813–824.

Groth-Marnat, G. (2000). Visions of clinical assessment: Then, now, and a brief history of the future. *Journal of Clinical Psychology, 56*(3), 349–365.

Haba-Rubio, J. (2005). Psychiatric aspects of organic sleep disorders. *Dialogues in Clinical Neuroscience, 7*(4), 335–346.

Han, E., & Liu, G. (2005). Racial disparities in prescription drug use for mental illness among population in U.S. *Journal of Mental Health Policy, 8*(3), 131–143.

Harrington, C., Gregorian, R., Gemmen, E., Hughes, C., Golden, K., Robinson, G., et al. (2000). *Access and utilization of newer antidepressant and antipsychotic medications.* The Lewin Group. Retrieved January 26, 2006, from http://aspe. hhs.gov/health/Reports/Psychmedaccess/chap01.htm.

Harvard Pilgrim Health Care. (2005). *Provider manual.* Retrieved June 24, 2005, from http://www.harvardpilgrim.org/pls/portal/docs/page/providers/manuals/med ical/C06-08_medicalmanage.pdf.

Hiatt, D., & Hargrave, G. (1995). The characteristics of highly effective therapists in managed behavioral provider networks. *Behavioral Healthcare Tomorrow, 4*(4), 19–22.

Hirschfeld, R. M., Williams, J. B., Spitzer, R. L., Calabrese, J. R., Flynn, L., Keck, P. E. Jr., et al. (2000). Development and validation of a screening instrument for bipolar spectrum disorder: The Mood Disorder Questionnaire. *American Journal of Psychiatry, 157*(11), 1873–1875.

Holder, H. (1998). Cost benefits of substance abuse treatment: An overview of results from alcohol and drug abuse. *Journal of Mental Health Policy and Economics, 1*(1), 23–29.

Hsich, L., & Kao, H. (2005). Depressive symptoms following ischemic stroke: A study of 207 patients. *Acta Neurologica Taiwan, 14*(4), 187–190.

Hunsley, J., & Bailey, J. (2001). Whither the Rorschach? An analysis of the evidence. *Psychological Assessment, 13*(4), 472–485.

Joint Commission on Accreditation of Heathcare Organizations. (2005). *About us.* Retrieved December 28, 2005, from http://www.jcaho.org/about+us/jcaho_facts.htm.

Jones, E. (2005, November). *Measuring the effectiveness of behavioral health interventions.* Paper presented at the New York Business Group on Health's Mental Health Benefits: Maximizing Quality and Outcomes Conference, New York.

Kaintz, K. (2002). Barriers and enhancements to physician-psychologist collaboration. *Professional Psychology: Research and Practice, 33*(2), 169–175.

Kanapaux, W. (2004). The road to integrated care: Commitment is the key. *Behavioral Health Tomorrow, 13,* 10–16.

Katon, W., Russo, J., & Von Korff, M. (2002). Long-term effects of a collaborative care intervention in persistently depressed primary care patients. *Journal of General Internal Medicine, 17*(10), 741–748.

Katon, W., Von Korff, M., & Lin, E. (1995). Collaborative management to achieve treatment guidelines: Impact on depression in primary care. *Journal of the American Medical Association, 273,* 51–58.

Katon, W., Von Korff, M., & Lin, E. (1997). Collaborative management to achieve depression treatment guidelines. *Journal of Clinical Psychiatry, 58*(1), 20–23.

Keefe, R., & Hall, M. (1999). Private practitioners' documentation of outpatient psychiatric treatment: Questioning managed care. *Journal of Behavioral Health Service and Research, 26*(2), 151–170.

Keyes, C. (2001). Risk management issues for clinicians who treat suicidal patients in managed systems. In J. Ellison (Ed.), *Treatment of suicidal patients in managed care* (pp. 153–172). Washington, DC: American Psychiatric Press.

Klonsky, E. (2002). Valid inferences from invalid tests? *American Psychologist, 57*(11), 990.

Kolbasovsky, A. (2004). Anger and mental health in type 2 diabetes. *Diabetes and Primary Care, 6*(1), 44–48.

Kolbasovsky, A. (2005). A pilot project to address the behavioral health needs of people with diabetes. *Managed Care Interface, 18*(11), 47–53.

Kolbasovsky, A., & Reich, L. (2005). Overcoming challenges to integrating behavioral health and primary care. *Journal for Healthcare Quality, 27*(5), 34–38.

Kolbasovsky, A., Reich, L., Romano, I., & Jaramillo, B. (2005). Integrating behavioral health into primary care: A pilot study. *Professional Psychology: Research and Practice, 36*(2), 130–135.

Kotin, A. (2006, January 12). *Strategies to integrate medical and psychiatric therapy.* Presentation at the New York Business Group of Health's The Hidden Factor in Spiraling Health Care Costs: The Connection Between Mental and Physical Health, New York.

Krieg, F. (1997). Managed care: A brief introduction. *Communique, 26*(1), 1–4.

Kroenke, K., Spitzer, R., & Williams, J. (2002). The PHQ-15: Validity of a new measure for evaluating the severity of somatic symptoms. *Psychosomatic Medicine, 64,* 258–266.

Lewin, R. (1990). Managed care and the discharge dilemma. *Psychiatry, 53,* 116–121.

Lin, E., Von Korff, M., & Katon, W. (1995). The role of primary care physicians in patients' adherence to antidepressant therapy. *Medical Care, 33,* 67–74.

Lin, E., Von Korff, M., Russo, J., Katon, W., Simon, G., Unutzer, J., et al. (2000). Can depression treatment in primary care reduce disability? A stepped care approach. *Archives of Family Medicine, 10,* 1052–1058.

Link, B., Andrews, H., & Cullen, F. (1992). Reconsidering the violence and illegal behavior of mental patients. *American Social Review, 57,* 275–292.

Little, D., Hammond, C., Kollisch, D., Stern, B., Gagne, R., & Dietrich, A. (1998). Referrals for depression by primary care physicians: A pilot study. *Journal of Family Practice, 47*(5), 375–377.

Lustman, P. (1988). Anxiety disorders in adults with diabetes mellitus. *Psychiatric Clinics of North America, 11*(2), 419–432.

Lustman, P., Anderson, R., Freeland, K., DeGroot, M., Carney, R., & Clouse, R. (2000). Depression and poor glycemic control: A meta-analytic review of the literature. *Diabetes Care, 23,* 934–942.

MacArthur Initiative on Depression and Primary Care. (2003). *Depression and primary care.* Retrieved December 1, 2005, from http://www.depression-primary care.org/.

Magellan. (2004). *Provider focus.* Retrieved May 3, 2005, from www.magellan-provider.com/about/whats_new/providerfocus/news/archives.

Magellan Behavioral Health. (2006). *Medical necessity criteria.* Retrieved October 5, 2005, from www.magellan provider.com/providing_care/clinical_guidelines/mnc2006.pdf.

Magellan Behavioral Health. (2004). *Provider manual.* Retrieved November 1, 2005, from https://www.magellanprovider.com/forms/handbooks/2006hb_final.pdf.

Magellan Health Services. (2004). *Clinical practice guidelines for the treatment of adults with substance use disorders.* Retrieved June 24, 2005, from https://www.magellanprovider.com/providing_care/clinical_guidelines/clin_prac_guidelines/sajan05.pdf.

Mallinger, J., Fischer, S., Brown, T., & Lamberti, J. (2006). Racial disparities in the use of second-generation antipsychotics for the treatment of schizophrenia. *Psychiatric Services, 57*(1), 13–136.

Maltsberger, J. (2001). The formulation of suicide risk. In J. Ellison (Ed.), *Treatment of suicidal patients in managed care* (pp. 1–14). Washington, DC: American Psychiatric Press.

Maly, M., Costigan, P., & Olney, S. (2005). Contribution of psychosocial and mechanical variables to physical performance measures in knee osteoarthritis. *Physical Therapy, 85*(12), 1318–1328.

Managed Care Weekly. (2005). *General business issues: More MCOs may bring behavioral health services in-house.* Retrieved December 12, 2005, from www.aishealth.com/managedcare/genbus/mcwinhouse.html.

Marchesi, C., Brusamonti, E., Borghi, C., Giannini, A., DiRuvo, R., Mineo, F., et al. (2004). Anxiety and depressive disorders in an emergency department ward of a general hospital: A control study. *Emergency Medical Journal, 21*(2), 175–179.

McCord, E., & Brandeburg, C. (1995). Beliefs and attitudes of persons with diabetes. *Family Medicine, 27*(4), 267–271.

McDaniel, S., Belar, C., Schroeder, C., Hargrove, D., & Freeman, E. (2002). A training curriculum for professional psychologists in primary care. *Professional Psychology: Research and Practice, 33*(1), 65–72.

McLellan, A. (1997). Can the outcomes research literature inform the search for quality indicators in substance abuse treatment? *Appendix B: Managing managed care: Improvement in behavioral health.* Retrieved January 3, 2006, from www.nap.edu.

McLellan, A., Woody, G., Metzger, D., McKay, J., Durrel, J., Alterman, A., et al. (1997). Evaluating effectiveness of addiction treatments: Reasonable expectations, appropriate comparisons. In A. Egertson, D. Fox, & A. Leshner (Eds.), *Treating drug abusers effectively* (pp. 1–6). Malden, MA: Blackwell Publishers.

McNeil, G. (2000). The collaboration between psychiatry and primary care in managed care. *Psychiatric Clinics of North America, 23*(2), 427–435.

Mechanic, D. (1998). Managed care, rationing, and trust in medical care. *Journal of Urban Health: Bulletin of the New York Academy of Medicine, 75,* 118–122.

Mechanic, D. (1999). The state of behavioral health in managed care. *American Journal of Managed Care, 5,* sp17–sp21.

Meyer, G., Finn, S., Eyde, L., Kay, G., Moreland, K., Dies, R., et al. (2001). Psychological testing and psychological assessment: A review of evidence and issues. *American Psychologist, 56*(2), 128–165.

MHN. (2005). *Practitioner manual.* Retrieved August 2, 2005, from https://www.mhn.com/practitioner/content.do?mainResource=pracManual.

Miller, A., Johnston, C., Klassen, A., Fine, S., & Papsdorf, M. (2005). Family physicians' involvement and self-reported comfort and skill in care of children with behavioral and emotional problems: A population-based survey. *BMC Family Practice, 6,* 12.

Minino, A., Arias, E., Kochanek, K., Murphy, S., & Smith, B. (2002). Deaths: Final data for 2000. *National Vital Statistics Reports, 50*(15).

Monahan, J. (1995). *The clinical predictions of violent behavior: Crime and delinquency issues.* Newbury Park, CA: Sage Publications.

National Committee for Quality Assurance. (2004). *State of health care report.* Retrieved May 30, 2005, from http://www.ncqa.org/communications/sohc2004/antidepressant_medication.htm.

National Committee for Quality Assurance. (2005a). *NCQA overview.* Retrieved December 15, 2005, from www.ncqa.org.

National Committee for Quality Assurance. (2005b). *State of health care report.* Retrieved February 6, 2006, from http://www.ncqa.org/Docs/SOHCQ_2005.pdf.

Nelson, E., Maruish, M., & Axler, J. (2000). Effects of discharge planning and compliance with outpatient appointments on readmission rates. *Psychiatric Services, 51,* 885–889.

Nemeroff, C., Musselman, D., & Evans, D. (1998). Depression and cardiac disease. *Depression and Anxiety, 8*(Suppl. 1), 71–79.

Odden, M., Whooley, M., & Shlipak, M. (2005). Depression, stress, and quality of life of persons with chronic kidney disease. *Nephron Clinical Practice, 103*(1), c1–c7.

Olfson, M., Haven, C., Fireman, B., Weissman, M., Leon, A., Sheehan, D., et al. (1997). Mental disorders and disability among patients in a primary care group practice. *American Journal of Psychiatry, 154*(12), 1734–1740.

Oppenheimer, K., & Swanson, G. (1990). Duty to warn: When should confidentiality be breached. *Journal of Family Practice, 30,* 179–184.

Pacificare Behavioral Health. (2001a). *ALERT annual report.* Retrieved June 24, 2005, from www.pbhi.com/providers_public/practitionerManual/generalmanual.

Pacificare Behavioral Health. (2001b). *Provider manual.* Retrieved June 24, 2005, from http://www.pbhi.com/Providers_public/PractitionerManual/GeneralManual/PractMan_TOC.asp.

Pacificare Behavioral Health. (2005a). *Network news: Provider newsletter.* Retrieved November 16, 2005, from http://www.pbhi.com/Providers_public/NewsInformation/Wr/WesternRegion.asp.

Pacificare Behavioral Health. (2005b). *Provider manual.* Retrieved November 1, 2005, from http://www.pbhi.com/Providers_public/PractitionerManual/GeneralManual/PractMan_TOC.asp.

Pacificare Behavioral Health. (2005c). *Psychological testing policy.* Retrieved December 20, 2005, from www.pbhi.com/Providers_public/practitionermanual/generalmanual/practman_D09.asp.

Paddock v. Chacko, 552 So2d. 410 (Fla. Dist. Ct. App. 1988), review denied, 553 So2d. 168 (Fla. 1989).

Persoons, P., Vermeire, S., Demyttenaere, K., Fischer, B., Vandenberghe, J., Van Oudenhove, L., et al. (2005). The impact of major depressive disorder on the short and long term outcomes of Crohn's disease treatment with infliximab. *Ailmentary Pharmacology and Therapeutics, 22*(2), 101–110.

Peyrot, M., & Rubin, R. (1999). Persistence of depressive symptoms in diabetic adults. *Diabetes Care, 22,* 448–452.

Phillips, D., Christenfeld, N., & Glynn, L. (1998). Increase in U.S. medication-error deaths between 1983 and 1993. *Lancet, 351,* 643–644.

Piotrowski, C. (1999). Assessment practices in the era of managed care: Current status and future directions. *Journal of Clinical Psychology, 55*(7), 787–796.

Prins, A., Kimerling, R., Cameron, R., Oumiette, P. C., Shaw, J., Thrailkill, A., et al. (1999). *The primary care PTSD screen (PC-PTSD).* Paper presented at the 15th annual meeting of the International Society for Traumatic Stress Studies, Miami, FL.

Psychotherapy Finances. (2004). *What's the right way to get off an MCO panel?* Retrieved March 1, 2006, from www.psyfin.com/articles/040401.htm.

Psychotherapy Finances. (2000). New survey report. *Psychotherapy Finances, 26*(10). Retrieved December 15, 2005, from http://www.psyfin.com/Survey2005.asp.

Quinn, C. (2003). Detection of malingering in assessment of adult ADHD. *Archives of Clinical Neuropsychology, 18*(4), 379–395.

Reich, L., Jaramillo, B., Kaplan, L., Arciniega, J., & Kolbasovsky, A. (2003). Improving continuity of care: Success of a behavioral health program. *Journal of Healthcare Quality, 25*(6), 4–8.

Richters, J., Arnold, L., Jensen, P., Abikoff, H., Conners, C., Greenhill, L., et al. (1995). NIMH collaborative multisite, multimodal treatment study of children with ADHD. *Journal of American Academic Child and Adolescent Psychiatry, 34,* 987–1000.

Robinson, W., Geske, J., Prest, L., & Barnacle, R. (2004). Depression treatment in primary care. *Journal of the American Board of Family Practice, 18*, 79–86.

Rogers, R., Sewell, K., Martin, M., & Vitacco, M. (2003). Detection of feigned mental disorders: A meta-analysis of the MMPI-2 and malingering. *Assessment, 10*(2), 160–177.

Roter, D., Hall, J., & Aoki, Y. (2002). Physician gender effects in medical communication: A meta-analytic review. *Journal of the American Medical Association, 288*, 756–764.

Saakvitne, K., & Abrahamson, D. (1994). The impact of managed care on the therapeutic relationship. *Psychoanalysis and Psychotherapy, 11*, 181–199.

Sabin, J. (1991). Clinical skills for the 1990s: Six lessons from HMO practice. *Hospital Community Psychiatry, 42*(6), 605–608.

Sabin, J. (1992). The therapeutic alliance in managed care mental health practice. *Journal of Psychotherapy Practice and Research, 1*, 29–36.

SAMHSA. (2001). *National household survey on drug abuse.* Retrieved August 12, 2005, from http://www.drugabusestatistics.samhsa.gov/nhsda/2k1nhsda/vol1/toc.htm.

Schneider Institute for Health Policy. (2001). *Substance abuse: The nation's number one health problem.* Princeton, NJ: Robert Wood Johnson Foundation.

Scholle, S. (2005). NCQA behavioral health measurement efforts. *Journal of Managed Care Pharmacy, 11*(3), S9–S11.

Schouten, R. (1993). Legal liability and managed care. *Harvard Review of Psychiatry, 1*, 189–190.

Sciehotta, F., Scholz, U., Schwarzer, R., Fuhrmann, B., Kiwis, U., & Coller, H. (2005). Long-term effects of two psychological interventions on physical exercise and self-regulation following coronary rehabilitation. *International Journal of Behavioral Medicine, 12*(4), 244–255.

Shlian, D., & Shlian, J. (1995). Health care indemnity consolidation: Implications for physician executive careers. *Physician Executive, 21*(11), 5–7.

Silver, R. (2001). Practicing professional psychology. *American Psychologist, 56*(11), 1008–1014.

Snoek, F. (2002). Breaking the barriers to optimal glycemic control: What physicians need to know from patients' perspectives. *International Journal of Clinical Practice Supplement, 129*, 80–84.

Spicer, J. (1998). Coping with managed care's administrative hassles. *Family Practice Management.* Retrieved December 29, 2005, from www.aafp.org/fpml/9803000fm/cover.html.

Spitzer, R., Kroenke, K., & Williams, J. (1999). Validation and utility of a self-report version of PRIME-MD: The PHQ primary care study. *Journal of the American Medical Association, 282*, 1737–1744.

Stein, M., Roy-Byrne, P., McQuaid, J., Laffaye, C., Russo, B., McCahill, M., et al. (1999). Development of a brief diagnostic screen for panic disorder in primary care. *Psychosomatic Medicine, 61*, 359–364.

Stork, E., Scholle, S., Greeno, C., Copeland, V., & Kelleher, K. (2001). Monitoring and enforcing cultural competence in Medicaid managed behavioral health care. *Mental Health Service and Research, 3*(3), 169–177.

Substance Abuse Mental Health Services Administration. (2001). *Summary of findings from the 2000 National Household Survey on Drug Abuse* (National Household Survey on Drug Abuse Series: H-13, DHHS Publication No. SMA 01-3549). Rockville, MD: Author.

Swanson, J., Holzer, C., Gangu, V,. & Jano, R. (1990). Violence and psychiatric disorder in the community: Evidence from the epidemiological catchment area surveys. *Hospital Community Psychiatry, 41*, 761–770.

Tabor v. Doctors Memorial Hospital, 563 So2d. 233 (La. 1990).

Tarasoff v. Regents of the University of California, 551 P2d. 334 (1974).

Trude, S., & Stoddard, J. (2003). Referral gridlock: Primary care physicians and mental health services. *General Internal Medicine, 18*(6), 442–449.

Tuttman, S. (1997). Protecting the therapeutic alliance in this time of changing health-care delivery systems. *International Journal of Psychotherapy, 47*, 3–16.

United Behavioral Health. (2004). 2004 USBHPC psychological testing guidelines. Retrieved January 17, 2006, from http://www.ubhonline.com/html/psych Testing/pdf/USBHPCPsychTestGuidelines.pdf.

Unutzer, J., Katon, W., & Callahan, C. (2002). Collaborative care management and late life depression in the primary care setting: A randomized controlled trial. *Journal of the American Medical Association, 288*, 2836–2845.

Unutzer, J., Katon, W., Callahan, C., William, J., Hunkeler, E., Harpole, L., et al. (2002). IMPACT Investigators. Collaborative care management of later-life depression in the primary care setting: A randomized controlled trial. *Journal of the American Medical Association, 288*, 2836–2845.

U.S. Department of Health and Human Services. (1993). *Depression in primary care: Treatment of major depression* (Vol. 2 AHCPR Publication. No. 93-0551). Rockville, MD: Agency for Health Care Policy and Research.

U.S. Department of Justice. (2006). *Americans with Disabilities Act.* Retrieved April 1, 2006, from www.usdoj.gov/crt/ada/adahom1.htm.

U.S. Preventive Services Task Force. (2002). *Screening for depression: Recommendations and rationale.* Rockville, MD: Agency for Healthcare Research and Quality. Retrieved September 1, 2005, from http://www.ahrq.gov/clinic/3rdusp stf/depressrr.htm.

Utilization Review Accreditation Commission. (2005). *About URAC.* Retrieved December 28, 2005, from http://www.urac.org/about_main.asp?navid=about&pa gename=about_main.

Value Options. (2005a). *Provider manual.* Retrieved September 1, 2005, from www.valueoptions.com/provider.

Value Options. (2005b). *Psychological and neuropsychological testing.* Retrieved December 30, 2005, from http://www.valueoptions.com/provider/hand books/criteria/outpatient/adultphychologicaltesting.htm.

Value Options New Mexico. (2005). *Provider forum.* Retrieved September 5, 2005, from www.valueoptions.com/newmexico/provider/forums/1.

VanDeCreek, L. (2000). Risk management and Tarasoff duty to protect. *APA Continuing Education Course.* Retrieved September 6, 2005, from http://www. psychpage.com/learning/library/counseling/violentclients.htm.

Viglione, D., & Hilsenroth, M. (2001). The Rorschach: Facts, fictions, and future. *Psychological Assessment, 13*(4), 452–471.

Weathers, F., Huska, J., & Keane, T. (1991). *The PTSD checklist military version (PCL-M).* Boston: National Center for PTSD.

Weilburg, J., Stafford, R., O'Leary, K., Meigs, J., & Finkelstein, S. (2004). Cost of antidepressant medications associated with inadequate treatment. *American Journal of Managed Care, 10,* 357–365.

Weiner, I. (2000). Using the Rorschach properly in practice and research. *Journal of Clinical Psychology, 56*(3), 435–438.

Wells, K., Sherbourne, C., & Schoenbaum, M. (2000). Impact of disseminating quality improvement programs for depression in managed primary care: A randomized controlled trial. *Journal of the American Medical Association, 283,* 212–220.

White, B. (1997). Mental health care: From carve-out to collaboration. *Family Practice Management, 4*(8), 1–5.

Wolff, N., & Schlesinger, M. (2002). Clinicians as advocates: An exploratory study of responses to managed care by mental health professionals. *Journal of Behavioral Health Services and Research, 29*(3), 274–287.

Wolraich, M., Feurer, I., Hannah, J., Baumgaertel, A., & Pinnock, T. (1998). Obtaining systematic teacher reports of disruptive behavior disorders utilizing DSM-IV. *Journal of Abnormal Child Psychology, 26*(2), 141–152.

Wood, J., Garb, H., Lilienfeld, S., & Nezworski, M. (2002). Clinical assessment. *Annual Review of Psychology, 53*, 519–543.

Wood, J., & Lilienfeld, S. (1999). The Rorschach inkblot test: A case of over-statement? *Assessment, 6*(4), 341–352.

Wood, J., Lilienfeld, S., Garb, H., & Nezworski, M. (2000). Limitations of the Rorschach as a diagnostic tool: A reply to Garfield (2000), Lerner (2000), and Weiner (2000). *Journal of Clinical Psychology, 56*(3), 441–448.

Wood, J., Lilienfeld, S., Nezworski, M., & Garb, H. (2001). Coming to grips with negative evidence for the Comprehensive System for the Rorschach: A comment on Gacono, Loving, and Bodholdt; Ganellen; and Bornstein. *Journal of Personality Assessment, 77*(1), 48–70.

Wood, J., Nezworski, M., Garb, H., & Lilienfeld, S. (2001). The misperception of psychopathology: Problems with the norms of the comprehensive system for the Rorschach. *Clinical Psychology: Science and Practice, 8*, 350–373.

Wood, J., Nezworski, M., Stejskal, W., Garren, S., & West, S. (1999). Methodological issues in evaluating Rorschach validity: A comment on Burns and Viglione (1996), Weiner (1996), and Ganellen (1996). *Assessment, 6*(2), 115–129.

Yohannes, A., Roomi, J., Baldwin, R., & Connolly, M. (1998). Depression in elderly outpatients with disabling chronic obstructive pulmonary disease. *Age & Ageing, 27*(2), 155–160.

Zdanowicz, N., Janne, P., Gillet, J., Reynaert, C., & Vause, M. (1996). Overuse of emergency care in psychiatry? *European Journal of Emergency Medicine, 3*(1), 48–51.

Zhang, X., Norris, S., Gregg, E., Cheng, Y., Beckles, G., & Kahn, H. (2005). Depressive symptoms and mortality among persons with and without diabetes. *American Journal of Epidemiology, 161*(7), 652–660.

Zimmerman, F. (2005). Social and economic determinants of disparities in professional help-seeking for child mental health problems: Evidence from a national sample. *Health Service Research, 40*(5), 1514–1533.

Zur, O. (1999). The managed care free private practice kit: From fear and trepidation to joy and prosperity. *Insurance Free*. Retrieved June 26, 2005, from http://www.division42.org/MembersArea/IPfiles/IPFall99/InsFree/Zur.html.

Index

Page numbers in *italics* refer to tables.